THE SLEEP RECIPE
THAT WORKS

reprogram
your
sleep

TARA
YOUNGBLOOD

REPROGRAM YOUR SLEEP
The Sleep Recipe that Works

Difference Press, Washington, D.C., USA
© Tara Youngblood, 2021

ISBN: 978-1-68309-290-2

Cover Design: Nakita Duncan
Interior Book Design: Anna Zubrytska
Editing: Cory Hott

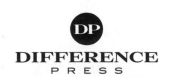

DIFFERENCE
PRESS

Advance Praise

"Research has clearly shown that sleep is critical for preventing disease and extending health span. But how do you get enough high-quality sleep in today's busy, modern world? That's exactly what Tara will show you how to do in this book. She translates the complex science on sleep into practical, actionable advice that will help you to find your optimal sleep recipe and 'reprogram' your sleep."

– Chris Kresser, founder of Kresser Intstitute for Functional & Evolutionary Medicine and author of New York Times bestseller *The Paleo Cure*

"You are holding a secret weapon, a manual to make nearly aspect of your life better. We cannot have a real conversation about your positions and tissue quality if this critical aspect of your life is out of whack. The solution is simple, start here."

– Dr. Kelly Starrett, coach/PT and two-time New York Times bestselling author

"I've trained over 150 high-level NBA players, and the blueprint to greatness all starts with sleep. I've never seen anyone more knowledgeable in the sleep game than Tara Youngblood. The way she unpacks the step-by-step process of how to become an optimized sleeper literally is not just a game changer for my NBA athletes, but it is a life changer for everyone who wants to get a great night's sleep – which would be everyone!"

– David Nurse, professional shooting
and skills trainer for NBA players -

To my family, for having to live with a walking sleep encyclopedia, and their support in writing this book. And to all the other people, like Susan, who need a path back to magical sleep.

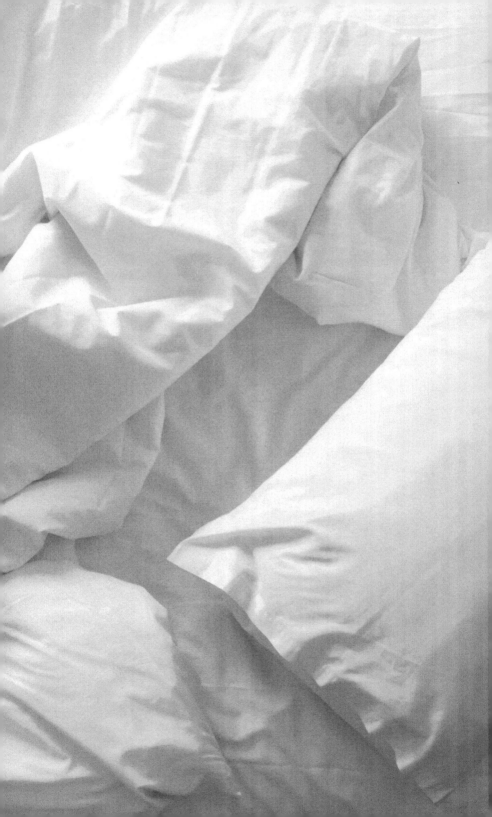

Table of Contents

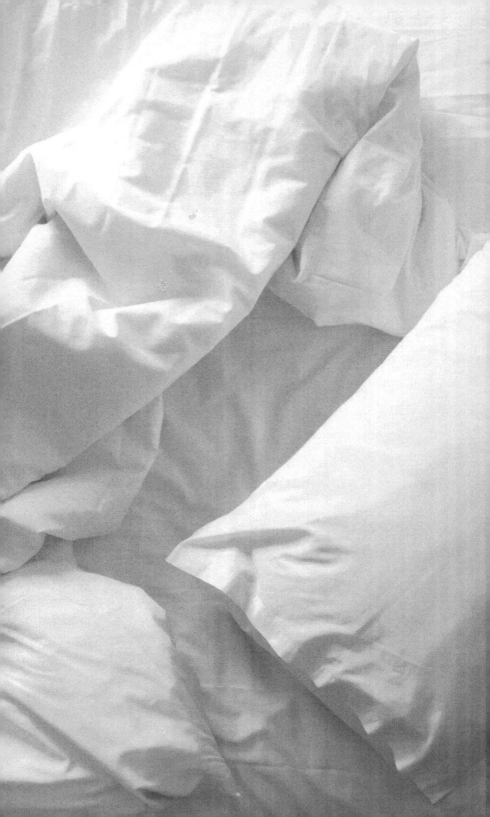

Foreword

I've always considered myself a pretty decent sleeper; no major complaints, and I usually wake up with a smile on my face and enthusiasm for a productive day – well, maybe after a cup of coffee. Over the past decade, the explosive growth of the primal/paleo/ancestral health movement has inspired me to study the subject of sleep further. It's clear that our modern sleep habits are one of the most offensive and health destructive disconnects in modern life – right up there with eating processed foods. I came to realize that my seemingly excellent sleeping habits and overall sleep effectiveness had tons of room for improvement. It's been a wonderful experience to further elevate my sleep game in recent years, and Tara Youngblood has been a great source of knowledge and inspiration to me in this area.

The thing about sleep is that it's ridiculously easy to right the ship and get an immediate payoff in the form of feeling fantastic, becoming sharper and more productive at work, improving workout performance and recovery, and having a happier disposition. Conversely, disrespecting the importance of sleep and being undisciplined with your sleep habits makes everything in life harder. There is plenty of research showing that even minor disturbances to your sleep cycles can cause a steep decline in both cognitive function, insulin sensitivity, and exercise performance and recovery.

There are definitely no excuses to making sleep number one on your list of healthy living objectives. While most everyone will acknowledge this, sleep seems to get too much lip service and not enough real action or behavior change. We also see a lot of misguided efforts and frustration when sleep challenges continue despite breaking your bank for a fancy new mattress or dutifully wearing blue-light blocking eyewear in the evening hours. It's time to right the ship with some simple, non-intimidating strategies that will help you prioritize sleep and make it easier to fall asleep gracefully, stay asleep, and cycle optimally through all the stages of sleep. The end result is that every day you will consolidate memories, hone powerful new neural connections, repair damaged cellular material to protect you from disease, and pop up every morning feeling refreshed and energized. The latter is one of our basic human rights that has been rudely compromised by the high-tech forces of modern life – particularly through excess artificial light and digital stimulation after dark.

I am pleased to welcome you to Tara Youngblood's new book, *Reprogram Your Sleep*, because it really is something special. Her story of loss, her struggle with extreme sleep deprivation and her passionate quest to discover real solutions will captivate you right away. I think you will greatly appreciate how Tara breaks things down and makes the science and strategy of sleep super simple: chunking sleep into three buckets and explaining how the often-overlooked variable of temperature (of both body and bed) is perhaps the single most important element of optimal sleep. Did you know we actually have a "sleep switch," and that temperature control is the gateway to becoming one of those sleep champions you envy when you seem them conking out seemingly at will on an airplane flight. These insights and more await you in this book, dense with scientific validation but in Tara's light-hearted, easy-to-read and easy-to-remember presentation

I've had the pleasure of working together with Tara and her husband Todd for several years with the burgeoning Chili TechnologyTM company, and I can attest that they are authentic and passionate in their dedication to helping you sleep better and live better. No matter how long you have struggled with sleep or how much you are convinced that your sleep peculiarities are genetic or inevitable, *Reprogram Your Sleep* offers hope as well as practical guidance. As you begin this book, I encourage you to relax, let the information soak in, and form empowering new beliefs that you can be that guy or gal who goes down gracefully and reliably every night and wakes up with a bounce in your step and a song in your heart.

Live awesome,
Mark Sisson
Miami Beach, Florida
January 2020

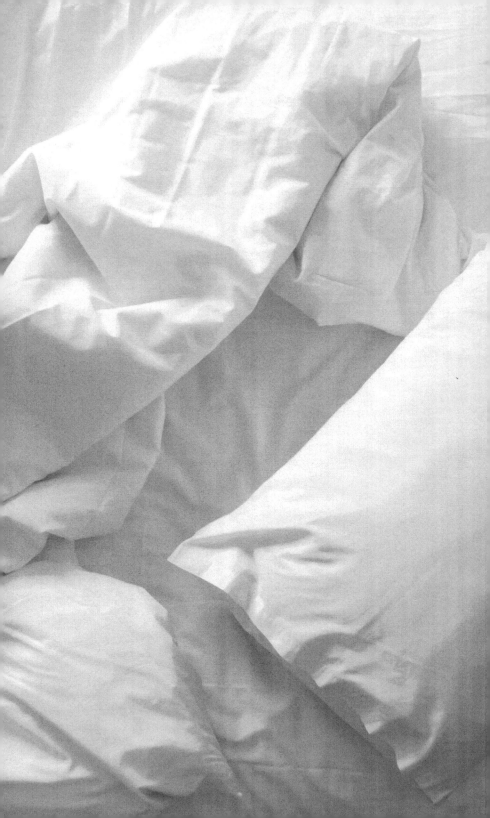

CHAPTER 1

Make the Impossible Possible

"The night is the hardest time to be alive and 4 a.m.
knows all my secrets."
– Poppy Z. Brite –

There is a great TED talk by RIVES, a poet. He describes 4:00 a.m. as an iconic moment that represents the worst of the night. In his talk, he shares a clip of Homer Simpson, who describes a mind-blowing thought that he could get whatever he wants, even at 4:00 a.m. He says, "Even on Christmas Day, four in the morning." Yes, even to Homer Simpson, 4:00 a.m.is the most surreal time to imagine doing anything. For me, 4:00 a.m. is the time when monsters roam the night, and I am one of those monsters – the un-sleepers, the zombies who wish for something else but are wandering their lonely landscape unable to sleep. Some will try to be productive; some just lie in bed; some search the internet, how you spend your sleeplessness is personal. Sleeplessness maybe from a trauma or part of depression. Whatever your reason for being at this point in your life, reading this book, you are ready to beat this sleeplessness and take back your life.

I met Susan in January; she is a successful businesswoman. She hadn't slept through the night in ten years and described getting up in the middle of the night as monstrous. We randomly met at a trade show. Her business and mine were not an immediate fit. She was from video production. I was peddling my product, the Chili-Pad. It is a sleep product so of course the subject of sleep came up. I believe that there are certain people in your life with whom you immediately connect. As a physicist, I would love to understand the energy flow between people better, but sometimes there is just magic. Susan and I had that; her pain felt like mine, and I needed to help her.

After the birth of her second child, Susan would wake up every night, dripping wet in sweat. Susan is a highly competent, successful wife, mother, and businesswoman. She would put towels under her body, have clean pajamas laid out. Nightly, she would take a shower and go back to bed. She wasn't in menopause. Many women experience this during menopause, but according to her doctors, there was nothing wrong with her. For those of you who are thinking it, no, this is not normal. It is not normal to wake up dripping in sweat unless you are working or standing out in the hot, humid southern summer.

The field of sleep science is still relatively small and new. But it is growing exponentially, thanks to both demand (the multifarious and growing pressures caused by the epidemic) and new technology (such as electrical and magnetic brain stimulators), which enables researchers to have what Matt Walker describes as "VIP access" to the sleeping brain. Matt Walker is probably best known for his book Why We Sleep. "Sleep medicine has only recently been recognized as a specialty of medicine. Its development is based on an increasing amount of knowledge concerning the physiology of sleep, circadian biology and the pathophysiology of sleep disorders. "Sleep research is in its infancy. Most of the information from the research has helped us learn more about sleep in specific categories.

Sleep Aid drugs like Ambien don't really help people sleep, they don't give good quality sleep. Insomniacs that don't want to take drugs are often left to find their own solutions."[1]

First, insomnia is the most commonly reported sleep-associated problem, affecting as much as 50 percent of the adult population periodically and 10 percent to 15 percent chronically.[2] Insomnia is defined as difficulty falling asleep, frequently waking up from sleep, waking too early and having trouble falling back asleep, or experiencing nonrestorative sleep. These problems occur despite whatever that person does to try to sleep and result in daytime sleepiness or fatigue and performance impairment. We suffer from it; animals suffer from it. It may seem to be as much a part of sleep as sleep itself. Why does it suck so bad then? Insomnia may have become part of your regular nightlife, but sleep is about habits. I want you to start thinking about how you form good habits and throw out bad ones. Everyone needs to start somewhere. This book starts with the basics on how to reset your sleep.

For Susan, every night was filled with waking up a hot, sweaty mess and every morning meant waking up exhausted. Her morning routine It started with coffee, watching some TODAY show, more coffee, and getting the kids breakfast and out the door. Her morning was about minimum viable activity, thought, and organization. It was totally about surviving. Susan would then work out. She has a healthy lifestyle. She works at home, when she can, and practices work-life balance as much as she can. She is a great person. She adopted another child and helps out in her husband's

---

[1] Walker, Matthew P. Why We Sleep: Unlocking the Power of Sleep and Dreams. Scribner, an Imprint of Simon & Schuster, Inc., 2018.

[2] Hare, Holly. "Lack of Sleep Is Killing Us, Experts Warn." *Orlando Sentinel*, 25 Sept. 2017.

business when she can. Being in the Insomnia Club wasn't going to limit her life. She wasn't going to fail. She doesn't give excuses.

But what does a life of poor sleep do to Susan behind the scenes? Is this something she can live with? Is getting by enough? When your doctor and gynecologist say you are fine, what can you do? Susan was getting only four or five hours of sleep. This amount of sleep is linked to cancer. When she doesn't sleep her natural killer cells – the ones that attack the cancer cells that appear in your body every day – drop by 70 percent. Does she know that lack of sleep is linked to cancer of the bowel, prostate, and breast or even just that the World Health Organization has classed any form of night-time shift work as a probable carcinogen? No, because we all do it: convince ourselves that those signs that something isn't right in our body are okay, that they will get better, that it can't last forever. But Susan lived without a solution for ten years. I have talked to many people where this is forty years or more, people who haven't slept through the night consistently since they were kids. I am guilty of the same excuses: "fake it till we make," "I will catch up later," "I am fine," "it is just stress, it will be better soon."

The little survivor voice is powerful. It is the voice for the inner strength that got Susan through her day. When I met Susan, she would not have looked, sounded or felt like someone suffering. She is and was a super high-energy, positive person. Having sleep issues is a mostly hidden weakness. Those of us in the Insomnia Club have perfected the art of getting by. But who stands up and says that the numbers are against you? More than twenty large-scale epidemiological studies all report the same clear relationship: the shorter you sleep, the shorter your life. Adults 45 years or older who consistently sleep less than 6 hours a night are 200 percent more likely to have a heart attack or stroke. With even just one night of modest sleep reduction your blood pressure will speed up, hour by hour, resulting in a significant increase in blood pressure.

As I said, Susan is outwardly healthy, but as we all know, health is hard to quantify outwardly. We are the products of our day-to-day lives, and things add up. Susan wasn't getting any deep sleep. There are basically three types of sleep: light, deep, and REM. Deep (or non-REM) sleep is much denser in the start of the night. In the second half of the night, it is much more REM sleep and your sleep cycles might not have any deep sleep. For you to fall asleep and stay asleep, your body has to drop two to three degrees Fahrenheit or one degree Celsius. Susan was not doing this, and she was not getting deep sleep.

When you look at our modern lives, it may stand out how completely obsessed with being comfortable we are. You may want light at the touch of a button. It has to be anytime, anywhere, cheap, and reliable. You want to be the ideal temperature and not sweat, hopefully ever, and if you do, it better be during a workout. You want to have information and data about everything whether you know how to use it or not – or even if it is good for you to hear about. Who doesn't listen to news? Popular news and gossip are driven by the train wrecks. When it comes to our "bedroom" – not sleep room, but bedroom – we don't skimp on modern luxury. Foams make us comfortable, and TVs help us relax. You may park your smart phones next to you everywhere you go, even while you sleep.

Susan isn't flashy or materialistic, but she is a modern American with a mattress to match. Foam is wonderfully comfortable, but we don't consider its thermal properties when we purchase it. When you buy mattresses online or sit on it in a mattress store, you are basically buying a couch for sleeping. When you sleep, your body is approximately at ninety-eight degrees Fahrenheit to start and puts off heat. That heat goes into the tiny bubbles of foam, and for the first few hours, the foam absorbs it. After that time, the foam hits maximum capacity and starts reflecting heat back to you. This would be great, except our bodies want to drop temperature while we sleep, and the lowest core body temperature is – you guessed it – in that magically surreal time between 2:00 and 4:00 a.m. (depending on when you start your sleep). Susan, whose body was clearly overheating during that time, was now hot. Sweaty, nasty mess hot. This wasn't her fault. Pregnancy hormones fluctuate a lot and can roller coaster after for a few months. Susan's hormones never reset.

Frequently finding yourself waking up drenched in perspiration: it's called night sweats. Also known as sleep hyperhidrosis, this condition involves repeated episodes of extreme sweating that can leave your sheets drenched. Night sweats differ from the occasional experience of waking up sweaty multiple times per night. In this case, following the sleep tip of setting your room temperature between sixty and sixty-eight degrees will not be enough. Sleep experts think that lower estradiol and higher luteinizing hormone levels were significantly correlated with indices of night sweats, especially in women. But for most of us, it means our body is thrown off. Hormones are not in check and the external/internal signals are way crossed.

I have heard stories of people over the years trying to solve this. It has ranged from multiple different mattress purchases to ice packs. Susan wanted to solve her monster problem herself so she would shower and quietly carry on. In one study it was estimated that 34 percent reported night sweats, one half of whom reported saturating their bedclothes. In another, it was as much as 41 percent.[3] Susan was clearly not alone. But when I sat down with

---

[3] Cooke, Rachel. 'Sleep Should Be Prescribed': What Those Late Nights out Could Be Costing You." *The Guardian*, 24 Sept. 2017.

her in January, she didn't feel like she had a solution. She didn't feel empowered. She felt alone, frustrated, and trapped with her nightly monster. It was a relatively simple and common problem, but Susan, a smart, capable person, was alone when she had it. The internet today is a wealth of information, but it can be hard to find the right solution. All the ingredients you need to sleep are laid out in an endless buffet. But how do you find what is right for you in that smorgasbord? Big Pharma puts Ambien and other sleep aids high in searches. Big mattress companies selling sleeping couches are also able to pay for top Google ad space. It is hard to be the CEO of your sleep and health.

Susan did not have a solution. But I did. Healing could begin. For her, it did start with temperature and a ChiliPad, but the journey only began there. In January and before, Susan and her husband would go to sleep after the last of the late-night talk shows. Not being good at something makes us put it off. We leave it to the end. Our weaknesses float down to the bottom of the list, and we like to pretend they don't exist. Insomniacs are well known for putting off sleep. Treating it like the misbehaving child that it is, we hope it will figure itself out in time out. We hope it will magically go away like it appeared, with the cause of the insomnia fleeing in the wake of us wanting sleep.

The first night of managing the temperature in her bed fixed the night sweats. No more sweaty monster appearances at 4:00 a.m. But sleep is complex. Temperature is just one part of a long list of tools you should have in your sleep toolbox. Chronotyping (your biological clock)[4], stress reduction mediations, gratitude, journaling, yoga, qigong, tai chi – the list is as endless as the internet.

---

[4] Korczak, A.l., et al. "Influence of Chronotype and Social Zeitgebers on Sleep/Wake Patterns." *Brazilian Journal of Medical and Biological Research*, vol. 41, no. 10, 2008, pp. 914–919., doi:10.1590/s0100-879x2008005000047.

But what that first sleep success did for Susan was magical. We all need a little confidence to take on our weakness, a success, a plan, a coach, something to get us to take a first step. This book is about finding that first step for you and arming you with the plan to take back control of your sleep and find out what you are capable of.

Seven months after I met Susan, we sat over a wonderful dinner. She was describing her morning now. It is full of buckets of energy. She still has coffee during the TODAY show, but she isn't curled up in her window seat, wrapped around the coffee. Coffee isn't the path to her day. She gets up and has done three to four things by the time she has the kids out the door. Her kids actually have asked why she is so focused and organized. She is productive an hour earlier than before and gets things done that could not fit on the list before. She has found more time. She has found more morning.

Susan's miraculous morning transformation begins with an all-new bedtime routine. The rather humorous part is that it has changed life for her husband as well. He was pretty skeptical in January and felt it was not a good idea at all. He is a contractor, a regular guy. He didn't see his sleep as a weakness. It is just a required part of the day – nothing special required of it or for it. Sleep just is sleep. They go to bed at 9:00 p.m. now. Sometimes they watch TV before bed there. Not everybody is going to follow sleep tips all the time. You will have to decide what will work for you long term. It is important, though, for the first thirty days to try to be as vigilant on your sleep and sleep interventions as possible. Just like managing a diet, you will find certain things are more important for your sleep. For Susan and her husband, it was timing and temperature that allowed them to win at sleep.

A recent study puts the evolutionary origin of sleep to somewhere around 450 million years ago. Study coauthor Philippe Mourrain, PhD, an associate professor of psychiatry and behavioral sciences at Stanford University, bases that claim on his work on zebrafish. According to Mourrain's work, zebrafish's sleep patterns indicate that sleep itself may have emerged along with the first vertebrates in the ocean. "Something that evolved so long ago and persists this long is testament to its importance,"[5] Mourrain adds. "The pervasiveness of these signatures speaks to a core function shared by all animals." You, like all the other animals, must learn to protect and push yourself to get great sleep.

"When I woke up this morning my girlfriend asked me, 'Did you sleep good?' I said, 'No, I made a few mistakes.'"
— Steven Wright

Sleep isn't new, and the problem of not sleeping isn't new. Marie de Manacéïne,[6] one of the first female physicians in Russia, was bothered by the complexity and unknown qualities of sleep: "We all love life, and we all wish to live as long as possible, but in spite of this, we sacrifice one-third, sometimes even half of our life in sleeping." In 1879, she began her quest to figure out what exactly sleep is, and she conducted the first sleep-deprivation experiment in animals.

It sounds horribly cruel: Marie kept puppies continuously awake, finding that they died after a few days of sleep deprivation. Over the years, sleep-deprivation experiments using other animals, like rodents and cockroaches, found similar fatal results. The cause of death in these cases, and how it relates to sleep, is still unknown. We do know we need sleep, the right sleep and at the right time.

It is amazing to sleep, to wake rested and feeling ready to start your day instead of your day slamming you awake with a loud

---

[5] Martineau, Pierre R., and Philippe Mourrain. "Tracking zebrafish larvae in group–status and perspectives." *Methods* 62.3 (2013): 292-303.

[6] de Manacéïne, Marie. "The physiology of sleep." (1897).

alarm. And it can be natural and easy. It can happen every night: sleep can be obedient. We sleep in the womb. As parents we quickly figure out how to "manage" our children's sleep. We know that if they don't get the sleep they need, they will be emotional monsters the next day. If we can apply the same motivations and processes that we apply to our children, we can ourselves be more successful at sleep. Yet we don't do the same for ourselves. For Susan, the reason she wanted sleep was there throughout her sleep problem. She didn't have an aha moment or epiphany. Doctors in her case kept telling her it was okay, and she had to keep looking herself to finally stumble on a solution. There is a phrase becoming popular in behavioral philosophy: your why. Identifying your why is about knowing what reasons motivate you. Your why can be because of your health or for your quality of life. For any diet or intervention that requires will, it is important to keep that why front and center. Everything gets hard sometimes, and it will be your why that keeps you going. For sleep, this is extra important because your mental state and willpower are extremely vulnerable when you aren't sleeping. You may need it on a stickie note on your mirror. My why was to spend better time with my kids, husband, and business. I wanted to be my best self, and sleep was preventing that. I needed to have a great sleep so I would be awake and happy when my boys climbed into bed to cuddle. I wanted them to start their day happy, and I needed my best me to do that. This sleep thing is absolutely beatable. Every single animal sleeps. It is an amazing function that we share with all other species. We are the only species that puts off sleep though. We fight it and disregard it. Your sleep is the time for your body to recover and for your brain to reset, file memories, and get healed and organized for another day. Animals may all sleep a little differently, but they all sleep. You may sleep differently than your spouse, or me, but we all can find our recipe for sleep.

CHAPTER 2

Finding My Recipe

*"I would enter your sleep if I could, and guard you there,
and slay the thing that hounds you, as I would if it had the
courage to face me in fair daylight. But I cannot come in
unless you dream of me."*

– Peter S. Beagle, *The Last Unicorn*

I joined the Insomnia Club as a child. My mother had to wear a hearing aid, so I learned quickly that calling out or making a big deal about sleep wasn't going to help. I got comfortable with the night – dragons, bad guys, shadows. Screaming didn't help. I needed to arm myself, buckle down and fix it, and if all else failed, turn on the light. I think this is why I became fascinated with the night, horror stories, and the witching hour. Our minds and imaginations are an important part of the sleep equation. We need to master the bad thoughts that crowd in after dark and beat them back. I still feel safer at dawn. My best sleep is still after the shadows are done. I guess I feel like the survivor at the end of a horror movie when the chaos of the night is lit up by the morning and it seems like it will be happily ever after. But I also learned to spend the extra time reading and researching. With the availability of technology, some people may spend their nights on their phones or computers, but for me it was reading books. But I found my way out of depression, sleeplessness, and exhaustion when I found my recipe for sleep. I had to own my sleep to beat it and make it work for me. Now that I know I can sleep when I want, I don't fear sleeping or put it off.

As a little girl, I wanted to be an astrophysicist. I loved the stars. In rural Alberta, there are lots of them, and the endless adventure of space called to me. But I also loved horses and animals and history, especially British history. I would fill up full of random facts. At fourteen, I became a lifeguard, and I loved saving lives. I worked at the YMCA, where there was almost a weekly incident of some kind. I was hooked. I got a chance to learn sports training while still in high school, and I also loved that. I think I fell in love with the idea of healing. I loved interacting with people who needed me. I learned that massage is about physically helping someone with your hands, but it is also about touch and energy, which is as much a part of the healing as the massage. I was the trainer for my husband's (Todd) football team in college. I like to think that taking care of sixty football boys prepped me for being the mother of all boys.

Those years as a trainer, I did tape ankles and fix cuts, but it was about giving the guys a loving connection. All people need hugs and love. Even five hugs a day will give you a healthy burst of oxytocin.[7] As a side soapbox, I think young men between the ages of sixteen and twenty-five are desperately in need of hugs. We need platonic caring relationships and a sense of community. There are multiple studies that show loneliness can increase mortality by 26 percent. Social media lets us feel like we are feeding that need to feel connected, but it is only skin deep. I think the relationships in

---

[7] Jessica, J. "Reasons Why You Should Be Hugging People More Often." (2018).

my sons' generation are much better at having platonic relationships. But I was able to be that mom/sister person for the teams I was a trainer for, and it was amazing, I like to think, for both sides.

I met Todd on the first day of college. He was an engineering major for three days with me before he switched to business. But as they say, it was all over by then, and we became partners. We did side hustles then; we were showing signs of entrepreneurial life already. After college, Todd got a job working for his uncle, Charles Hall. Crazy fact: he invented the waterbed. Yep, it was his master's thesis project. I was from Canada, and my student visa ended when I graduated. Work permit delays and lack of direction meant I became a jack of all trades as I struggled to find my career home.

Two years after starting work for his uncle, Todd's job moved us to Minnesota when Charlie sold the company. Young, broke, and hungry for adventure, we moved. But then, two years later, we moved again. We had Ty then, and it seemed like we were both trapped in a corporate maze. Ideas and business growth were often met with broken promises of bonuses. In 2000, we went out on our own. I started market research, and Todd worked the relationships at night and weekends until we got stable enough to jump two feet into the entrepreneurial life.

In 2001, Caleb was born, and we settled into this entrepreneurial life. We found our niche in helping Asian companies enter the US market. The factories were generally making a quality component and were looking to diversify into finished goods. I think this is where I got bit by the market analytics bug: finding new uses for these components, sizing up markets, and determining price, retailer, and packaging. We got to see and touch it all. But it is easy to want to chase something bigger, so when the opportunity to join another business in Charlotte came up, we jumped at it. Todd may not share my hunger for all types of knowledge, but business anything lights him up.

It didn't work. There were eleven partners and one lead partner. Quickly it became clear that the moral code we did business in and the company were not matched. Things were never illegal or obviously wrong to someone on the outside, but on the inside, they were fifty shade of gray for sure. We decided then that we would only do business that fit our moral standards. We will bend rules or even find ways around them when we need to, but not if there is a moral cost. We would not treat employees like disposable parts. And we couldn't sleep at night if it seemed like tax issues and other business rules were outside of what we felt was reasonable. We walked away. Living in Mooresville, with Samuel on the way, we started over. We were able to keep our clients and slowly worked to gain back a foothold. We would find a mesh of innovations from different markets and uses and combine them for others as consultants and ourselves for our own products.

Benjamin was born in December 2006. It felt like our family was complete. We had our tribe of four boys. Todd's parents had retired from New York and were living nearby. It seemed like we were well on our way to the picture-perfect American life.

Benjamin was a healthy baby. Smiley, he liked to watch his brothers. At the end of May 2008, he seemed to get a bad ear infection. We took him to his doctor and a night later to urgent care. Then over the weekend, we had to go to the emergency room. He seemed to be in so much pain, and nothing helped him. In the early morning, he started having seizures. We rushed him to the emergency room. At that time, they did a spinal tap, which showed he had bacterial meningitis. We still had the other boys at home, so I went with Benjamin.

When trauma happens in your life, you can remember every vivid detail. I still can smell the disinfectant and the ticking of the clock. I would pump great milk for my baby who would never wake up. In twenty-four hours, the meningitis dissolved his brain. After talking with the doctor and learning it was not going to get better, I went to sit in the hallway. A wonderful nurse woman came and scooped me up in a hug. She asked if I wanted her to pray with me. In that moment, it was clear to me that I didn't need to pray for him. He was everything he needed to be. We chose for him to be an organ donor. Our little boy saved two lives. It is extremely rare for a child at Benjamin's age to be a donor. Usually disease is not kind to a little body, but it had been so fast for him that only his brain was damaged.

I think when we look at what makes a life meaningful, it is how we can leave the world a little bit better than when we came into it. I want to say that the world was changed for the better because I was born. We often use time as a measurement in how good a life was. Benjamin made an impact for those families. He was the answer to their prayers. He could have lived sixty years but never done that. We said goodbye to our little Boop-Boop.

I was always a visual, romantic, and idealistic person. We lived the American dream, living in suburbia. We had a successful business and four beautiful boys, but that bubble was suddenly burst. We were broken, not beautiful. Dads and moms, men and women, people grieve differently. But there isn't room for grief during the day with three boys shocked in the reality of death. There isn't room for grief when you run your own business. There isn't bereavement leave for us. My sleep disappeared. Todd buried his anger, and we moved on.

Depression is a horrible thing. It is so easy to hide from the outside world. I wasn't sleeping, which has a comorbid relationship with depression. When you are depressed, you can't sleep, and if you can't sleep, you get depressed. I roamed our house hoping that if I lay in one of the kid's beds or on the couch, I would find sleep. Mostly, I curled up in my closet and tried to hide.

There have been studies that show, as humans, we can detect loneliness in each other. Unfortunately, the reaction is to turn away from that person. Before Benjamin's death, I was part of Bible studies and friend groups, but after, suddenly, I wasn't included anymore. The depression got worse before it got better.

In 2008, we had Hadyn. I felt that it was important we found a way to be a family of four, just with a constant fifth angel. During the pregnancy and first few months, we all held our breath. The boys had been weird around other people's babies as they grieved; they needed to heal. Hadyn was the glue that knit our family back together. But the rest of the tsunami was still arriving.

In a period of a year, we lost Todd's dad, and the business was hit with a malicious patent lawsuit. It was about pool floats. We didn't have a great attorney; they had sharks. We struggled to pay the endless legal bills. They sued businesses like us for a living. The patent wasn't theirs. We had prior art, but we lost. Chalk one up to business IQ. But the stress suffocated us. Sleep was not something I could win at. Sleep was impossible, and it was quickly becoming a health issue.

At the same time, Todd and I explored the idea of bringing a temperature sleep product to market. We had developed as market niche specialists. Sleep seemed up and coming with Select Comfort and Tempurpedic selling ultimate sleep comfort as pressure. But pressure was not the problem for us. Todd has always slept hot. Even our boys all sleep hot. I would arm myself against the heat with piles of pillows and blankets. We saw the need for temperature adjustment for the bed. If you could adjust temperature for a driver and a passenger in a car, then we felt like it made sense to do that in a bed as well. ChiliPad was born.

The idea was that I could be warm and snuggly when I climb into bed and Todd could get his side to be as cold as possible. Picture a slab of ice. Getting into my warm and snuggly bed, it would still take me an hour or more to fall asleep. Then I would wake up a few hours later, stare over at Todd sleeping comfortably and I desperately wanted to win at sleep. My body and emotions felt broken.

My grandmother was German, from Munich. Her father was the head of the Department of Justice when Hitler came to power. He did not agree with Hitler, and so he was one of the first to disappear. My great-grandmother opened a boardinghouse to survive. Before the war started, my grandfather would travel for Barclay's Bank, and he stayed at her boardinghouse. He met my grandmother while staying there, and they fell in love and moved back together to South Africa. He left for war against Germany three months later. My grandmother spoke only German. She was pregnant with my dad when she lived on my grandfather's family farm outside of Johannesburg. She was utterly alone.

Fortunately, there was a nun who spoke some German, and she came to help my grandmother delivery the baby. Raising my dad for the next four years alone was everything you could imagine. Farming can be tough with today's equipment and modern infrastructure. She raised Jack Russel terriers so there was always a dog around my dad to keep the snakes away from him. She fixed water pumps and God knows what else to keep that farm going. She got it to thrive. She didn't have anyone to solve her problem. She had to research and find her own solutions to her problem.

I had to find a solution. My aha moment came while I was at a trade show in Las Vegas. When we first sold the ChiliPad, it was to retailers. Surrounded by mattress companies, pillow sales guys, and vendors touting the sleep they would give made me feel hypercritical. I hadn't mastered sleep. How could I possibly sell it to someone else? Buying a new mattress, pillow, or even the Chili-

Pad may help some people, some of the time, but it hadn't totally helped me. I believe magic happens when there is a recipe and a process. I thought of my grandmother and how she had to solve her problems. I had to dive deeper to define a sleep recipe.

Over the years of selling ChiliPad, we have had people come to us with amazing stories of how this simple temperature thing had changed their life. The list of professional athletes, celebrities, and other VIPs is incredible. From royalty to former presidents, people were using temperature to manage their sleep. But although it was apparently working for all of those people, and there is real science in how temperature helps sleep, it wasn't able to fix me. Sleep and health are not a simple equation. We are a sum of our genetics, our experiences, and our lives. The only person who can test and prove what works is ourselves.

I had to define the variables in sleep. Over three hundred books and literally thousands of research papers later, I was starting to shape a picture of sleep. My nice warm bed was great to fall asleep, but it was actually hurting me in the middle of the night. When I cooled things down, I was too cool in the morning. I searched for and found the biological triggers for sleep and sleep states and dug into how far I could take temperature and my sleep.

I put my bed up on risers, put sensors in the bed, next to the bed, and on me. I tried to keep the science lab managed under the bed risers, but there were generally cords everywhere. I had hyper-thermia machines, medical pads, use packs. I had PEMF magnets in my bed and sound machines generating all frequencies. I had mats with crystals and supplement bottles covering my bathroom counter. I may be Amazon's best customer. I think I own and have tried everything in the sleep category.

I have never been someone who would be described as a specialist. I am good at lots of things but in general not great at any one thing. I am addicted to books and knowledge in an almost unhealthy way. But I do feel like my gift is tracking patterns, connections, and clusters. I think in what computer scientists like to call complex networks. Our bodies and minds are the best manifestations of this network. Nodes are connection points, and super nodes are what they sound like: bigger connections. These recipes are a guide for you to make the connections in your body, mind, emotions, and life. I will share the patterns and possible connections. What are your must-have rules? What are things that help but can be flexible? What delivers you sleep and health? What makes your recipe repeatable? Most importantly, what gives you your why? For me, it was being awake and happy to spend time with my kids, husband, and even be better at work. Start defining why you need to do this: it will lift you up when it gets hard.

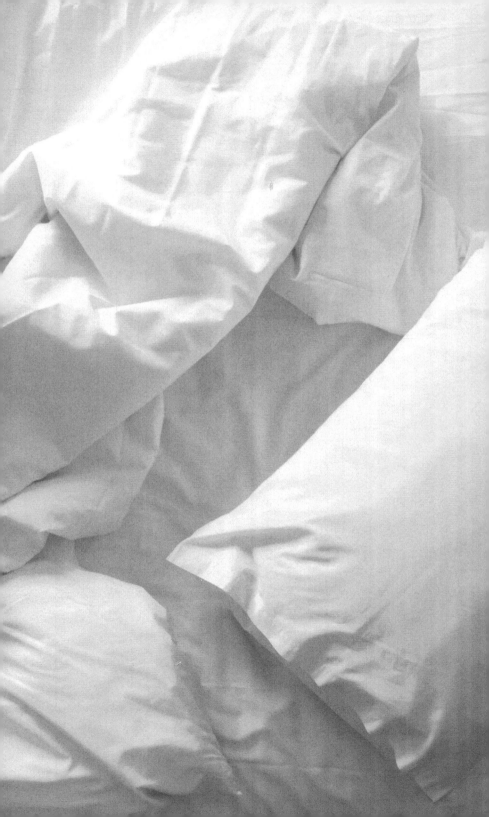

CHAPTER 3

What Is a Sleep Hacker Anyway?

"What we fear doing most is usually
what we most need to do."
— *Timothy Ferriss, The 4-Hour Workweek* —

The first biohacker I ever followed was Tim Ferriss. He was instrumental in putting ChiliPad on the map. I followed him for his four-hour workweek and four-hour body books. He was a big part of my inspiration to try some experiments to get a sleep recipe that would make my body be what I wanted it to be. I haven't perfected everything, not even close, but I think my sleep process is worth a try and this is where we are going in this chapter. By the end, I expect you to have a good idea what your recipe will look like. The essence is clearly defining the required outcome and measuring its effectiveness. You must love yourself and your why enough to continue to evolve your sleep journey. Hack yourself, your mind and your body to find your triggers for success.

Self-Inventory

Terri was one of our early users. She was an Ob/Gyn and in the peak of menopause. She saw people in her practice who suffered from hot flashes, but she couldn't solve it for herself. She didn't want to take hormones or the other therapies her fellow doctors prescribed, but she was miserable. When we met her, she had just bought a new mattress to "help" her sleep better. It was a top-of-the-line memory foam version. It only made it worse. She slept in the spare room so her husband could still sleep. It was in the early days of our e-commerce business, but she found us. The ChiliPad changed her life. It reduced and almost eliminated hot flashes at night and cut them in half during the day. We agreed that the bonus daily reduction had more to do with great sleep, but she was thrilled with the bonus.

Terri had bought a mattress to fix her problem, but it wasn't the right solution. When there are problems in our sleep. We have to understand how they fit together before we can actually solve it. The goal with this program is to spend less time and money, experiment with what works, and then refine your plan. The self-inventory step is important. Dive in and find out what is going on in your sleep. You are your best chance at figuring out what is going on, so be honest and spend the most time on this step.

Putting Your Sleep into Buckets

Ten thousand hours and hundreds of sleepless nights led me to I discover what I like to call the three buckets of sleep. Why buckets? Well, it may be the farm girl in me. Messy stuff goes into buckets. There are baskets and buckets to collect shoes and miscellanies around our house. I like to organize things that way; mostly I like to make science more lovable, and simple visualization seems to help people to like it better. Physics is not lovable, so I had to adapt early. The thing to keep in mind is that the buckets are not equal and may not be equally weighted for you. When you start to put your problems into these buckets of time and sleep, you may find that some of them, like stress, can go into all of the buckets. Things like stress are going to need to be managed all day and in each sleep bucket. See why it is messy?

The buckets are really windows of time. Each time you go through the window of time you complete the bucket and move to the next. When you pass each end point of the bucket, something changes in your body. Just like passing the numbers on a big twenty-four-hour clock, your body mechanisms are on a timer. We have our own body clock, who knew? This is your circadian rhythm. They are endogenous (built-in, self-sustained, self-propelled); they are adjusted or entrained to the local environment. Back to you running laps in the training pen. As you pass by certain things, they will trigger you. You see something; you will respond. Those external cues are called zeitgebers[8] (from German, literally "time giver"). Key points of interactions are light, temperature, and redox cycles.

Redox cycles are fascinating, well maybe to me and a small collection of others, but just in case you want a touch more information: Oxidation-reduction reactions are essential to life as the core mechanisms of energy transfer.[9] They occur when an electron is lost by one substance and is transferred to another. The cycle of this transfer happens in conjunction with our twenty-four-hour clock. Why does this matter? Redox reactions are everywhere. Your body uses redox reactions to convert food and oxygen to energy, plus water and carbon dioxide, which we then exhale. The batteries in your electronics also rely on redox reactions, because your body, just like batteries, needs to transfer energy from one place to another, like your battery in your flashlight transferring the power needed to light up the bulb. You are part of an energy cycle, and this cycle is timed to your biological clock.

---

[8] Monk, Timothy H. "Enhancing circadian zeitgebers." *Sleep* 33.4 (2010): 421-422.

[9] Bothwell, Mia Y., and Martha U. Gillette. "Circadian redox rhythms in the regulation of neuronal excitability." *Free Radical Biology and Medicine* 119 (2018): 45-55.

Pretty important stuff, and it all uses this clock inside us for the timing of why, when, and how. We all have our own, but mine may not be the same as yours. This is called a chronotype. Our bodies measure time slightly differently. We are kind of running on different time zones. Dinner is still dinner in the United Kingdom and the United States, but we time it differently. Again, fancy fact, but how does this help you sleep? If we are running around that lap ring and we miss the timing window for sleep, we miss out on all the other things that are happening in our bodies to help with sleep. We need to learn to listen to this inner clock and respect its timing so we can time our hacks better.

Combining chronotype, basically the timing of sleep elements based on the circadian rhythm, with temperature that matches what the body is doing naturally at that time creates the basis for a magical sleep recipe. Adding healthy habits, thoughts, and processes that give your body the best framing for sleeping, changes sleep into a consistently amazing experience.

The first bucket is the sleep switch. This phrase was first coined by Clifford Saper from Harvard.[10] The ventrolateral preoptic nucleus (VLPO) is a small cluster of neurons in the hypothalamus that are the center of the brain's sleep mechanisms. The sleep switch means the VLPO neurons in our brains are triggered to tell us to sleep. Cool? Yes, exactly. It is a change of temperature that causes them to release melatonin and cause sleep. Awesome. I would like to flip a switch to sleep. This is a switch that when we are running our laps, we want to know and respect. Ignoring the switch and putting off sleep can make it much more difficult later.

But how do I flip the switch as I run by during my day? It requires change. When you think about our lives today and the

---

[10] Saper, Clifford B., et al. "Sleep State Switching." *Neuron*, vol. 68, no. 6, 2010, pp. 1023–1042., doi:10.1016/j.neuron.2010.11.032.

constant comfort temperature environment, there is no change. Even a hundred years ago, we lived more entrained to the temperatures outside. Today, our modern conveniences allow us to have light and temperature be constant. We can always be the same. There isn't a sunset with a corresponding temperature drop and the cool breeze swirling around us in the early evening. We need to trigger that switch. Light can also switch on sleep. But just like there is generally not a cool breeze in our living room, the sun doesn't set inside our houses. We start our day with our phones, TV, lights, and computer and end it that way as well. There is no change to flip our switch — more on that later. There is a theme to this hacking thing.

First, change isn't bad. Our bodies are looking for it. And to recognize that change might mean not being comfortable all of the time. We need to push ourselves out of our comfort zone and into the space where we flourish — change. In the first bucket, we need to change our minds to relax, unwind, and destress and be grateful, peaceful, and loving, receiving and giving hugs. Change your temperature, take a bath or shower, or go for a walk. Think about what causes your body to experience a ten-degree temperature shift. We need to change our lighting to dim. Think of sitting around a campfire. Let yourself relax. Turn off the LEDs and light a candle.

In 2016, music producer Rick Rubin, unbeknownst to us, was an avid user of our product. He and some other biohacker, Paleo, Keto, and health people joined us to help elevate ChiliPad. We met at Mark Sissan's house in Malibu, founder of Primal Kitchen and Mark's daily apple. Mark is an investor in Chili. Mark's wife had just installed energy-efficient LEDs everywhere. Rick is so humble and unassuming, but he did not approve of the LEDs, so we had our business meeting sitting crisscrossed in front of the fireplace with the sun setting outside — absolutely a Zen experience and a far cry from a stiff and over-illuminated boardroom. You don't need all of that light at night. Light more candles or share time in front of the fireplace. I can hear Todd's voice saying that romantic time is always good advice, and yes, it actually is.

Managing Our Day to Control Our Night

You can see pictures of pets cuddling all over the internet. Humans are pack animals. We get bursts of oxytocin from hugs and physical contact. Is cuddling part of your routine? Animals count too. My dog, Nina, and three cats wait for me to settle in the evening. If it is a good night and all of my boys are home, we all cuddle on the bed. You're never too old or too big to cuddle. We got a king-sized bed and reinforced it to handle all of us. But nothing feels better in the world. Nothing makes your body relax like sharing space.

I have to govern this time. Todd and I have different habits in the evening. I need to clear my head and not think about work if work is stressful or not think about kid stuff if there is kid stuff going on. I need to let the day go. Todd wants to talk about his day while I want to wind down. He has issues he wants to get off his chest. I think some of the worst were business cashflow problems. There's nothing like saying, "Not sure how we are going to make payroll this week" and then shutting off the lights. I would then immediately want to get up and fix the problem instead of sleeping, and I often did. Then I would want to pounce on him first thing in the morning with my solution; he wasn't pleased to talk business first thing. We struggled with this before we made rules about it. Being a hacker can be as simple as making rules for yourself and, in this case, for your relationship before and after sleep.

Heather and I first connected over Facebook. She was an avid ChiliPad user. Since her early twenties, she hadn't sleep through the night. The ChiliPad settled down her temperature and helped her sleep. She would routinely comment that she would give up her Chili-Pad before her husband. Makes me want to add an LOL emoji. She was sure that she needed it set super cold in order to sleep because she had woken up hot for so long. The ChiliPad is like an old-fashioned thermostat: once you set it, it stays that way. She was too cold at bedtime. She also hung out and watched TV in bed, with the lights on, while drinking a glass of wine. Remarkably she was having a hard time falling asleep. She needed some new rules to set the right habits for bedtime, not just the ones that she had always done.

Heather needed to reset bedtime, even though she had solved the biggest problem that was waking her up at night. She had to tidy up bedtime. She found she could compromise and still watch TV but had to dim the lights, nix the wine, and set the ChiliPad to start to cool only when she was truly about to sleep. That way, lying in bed while watching TV got her bed warm and snuggly for falling asleep. The ChiliPad takes about twenty to thirty minutes to go from all the way warm to cool. Heather just needed to prewarm her bed. Then while she was winding down, she was warm. The warm bed allowed her to relax, but when she was turning off the lights, she would turn down the temperature to get the temperature right for deep sleep. Don't accept that what you are doing today is okay. You may need to be flexible to get your best sleep.

This happens for diet and exercise routines as well. I have to set ground rules to not sabotage myself and be clear with the people around me. It sucks to be offered cake or some other banned treat when you diet. People are not always supportive when you are trying to grow and evolve. People are much more interested when you are needy. By changing yourself to be a sleep hacker and not an insomnia sufferer, you are a sleep conqueror.

My favorite book, possibly of all time, *Shantaram,* is about overcoming unbelievable difficulties, survival and perseverance.

"It took me a long time and most of the world to learn what I know about love and fate and the choices we make, but the heart of it came to me in an instant, while I was chained to a wall and being tortured. I realized, somehow, through the screaming in my mind, that even in that shackled, bloody helplessness, I was still free: free to hate the men that were torturing me, or to forgive them. It doesn't sound like much, I know. But in the flinch and bit of the chain, when it's all you've got, that freedom is a universe of possibility. And the choice you make, between hating and forgiving, can become the story of your life."

To me, sleep hacking – choosing to own my body and my health – is this freedom. In the middle of the night, insomnia feels like it has chained you to the wall and is beating the will out of you, to succeed, to overcome, to just get dressed and make your bed in the morning.

I decided to break the emotional chains around sleep, you have to decide to forgive yourself for failing at sleep. You must find your compass, drive, beacon. You must climb a mountain and you need to start with your why.

If you can, I would find a place – a grassy patch in the middle of a park, your backyard, the beach, a mountain top. You know what that place is for you. Go there, get barefoot, make sure your body connects to the earth. Now, just be.

Shantaram is literally chained in a basically empty room with every human necessity striped away. There isn't anywhere for your soul to hid. This is where you can find your most unique self. What makes you and only you, you? Warrior, Defender, Good and Bad, Black and White. There is something in that room that can't be stripped away. Something no one can take from you.

Yes, it maybe the bad experiences that scar us and shape the glasses that we see the world through. But everyone has a basic sense of what their soul looks like. For me, it has always been simple. I have a high pain tolerance and am not afraid of dying, but I am driven to always do the right thing. I may not always get everything right, but I want to. In my head, my image and code are defined by a particular scene because it added clarity for me.

In this scene, I am in Germany at the start of World War II. I have a moment where I need to decide to save my life or stand up to the soldiers demanding I turn over my Jewish friend. I choose death. I understand that it probably means we both die. I understand that many people lived through such a scene and then saved many more lives by not dying in that moment. But I can't. I am not suicidal in this scene. I want to live but not at the cost of not doing what is true to my soul. I would break trust with the sacred part of me.

I am so grateful I have never had to choose like that, but that trust bond with my soul defines me. As I constantly battle to remind myself, through writing this book, I am standing up against this battle of sleep. I am not a person who shares what I have shared as part of this process. I am a solid introvert. But when I sleep, I want to stand up for what is right and help people escape from what is oppressing them. This is my pact with my soul.

What is something that you could not break for yourself? What is your most sacred principle? This is your gift to the universe. This is what you are not able to share to the fullest when you are chained down by insomnia. You and only you can find it. It is not required to follow this plan. Nobody but you will know if you have defined this for you. But it is a special key to unlocking your will.

It is likely that this piece of you has been buried and unkept. But it is the key to understanding your superpower, your dream come true. When your brain is low on energy or someone is sabotaging your plan, this is the superpower that when activated will pull you through.

When I am tired, I want to withdraw and give up. Your bio-chemistry of being exhausted, depressed, and weary is strong, but this kernel of you can shine through that. Human beings are incredibly resistant. You can keep going well past when our bodies should stop. It is this kernel that allows for that miracle.

I had to manage my day to control and conquer my grief and depression. I had to manage the when and how of my day. Intermittent fasting is a huge fad at the moment, and to me, it fits with our biological clocks. Match your day to your chronotype and the buckets of sleep work so much better.

Organizing Your Sleep and Health

Being a hacker isn't just about knowing your recipe and hacking your system of sleep. It is about shifting the definition of who you are to that kernel of truth and then creating the physical recipe that brings that kernel to life. The superpower, the world needs is the strength and the purpose to get you past chains and pain. Pulling all of this information is tough. I am building an app to help with this process because there is a lot of information here. Look at the sample days and map your day to those. I used an Excel spread-sheet for a while to plug in when to do what during the day. Your self-inventory put the right things in the right buckets at the right time and rechecking that inventory keeps it organized. You may feel overwhelmed but hang tight. You have only begun the ride.

CHAPTER 4

Kryptonite versus Superpowers

"If I had to choose one superpower, it would not be wisdom, money, love, friendships; it would be sleep because a great sleep gives you all of those wrapped up in a bow of a happy and peaceful mind."

— Tara Youngblood —

When I think about where I am today, in life, in my sleep, it is all about the whys. When I think about the areas I am still working on, I believe it is because my whys haven't gotten big enough to convince me to put in the effort to change. I feel like sleeping gives my brain, my body, and my soul room to do the things I want to in a day. I have bigger dreams and accomplish bigger to-do lists with sleep. It is easy to focus on your weaknesses, your kryptonite. But what is your gift? What superpower is uniquely yours? I have had some people, like Aaron, who spiritually dug into this idea. He asked himself what God wanted him to do. He needed sleep to be the pastor he was led to be. He could reach out more and love his congregation more if he was a happy, healthy, and had great sleep. I will probably say it many more times but find your why and your superpowers will be waiting.

Health outcomes in our modern society are no longer about surviving; being healthy is about managing your health. Aaron was a thirty-seven-year-old guy who looked healthy on the outside. When he asked his doctor, his doctor said he was good. But he wasn't. Sleep is a big part of your health equation. "No aspect of our biology is left unscathed by sleep deprivation,"[11] as Matt Walker said. When we don't sleep well, we have a higher risk of mortality, Alzheimer's and memory problems, and chronic disease. Sleep is the difference between living well and have good quality of life until the end. For Aaron, it is the difference between just doing his job and, as he says it, "doing God's work."

Still it may be difficult to understand how sleep is such a critical part of health outcomes. Alzheimer's and loss of cognitive function becomes a big fear for us all as we age. We all dread the nursing home, where our body is technically alive, but our mind is gone. Every night your brain, during deep sleep, in essence, gets a car wash. Our spinal fluid flushes out toxins[12] and keeps our brains free of buildups. If we don't sleep, that doesn't happen.

In basic terms, Alzheimer's is related to the amyloid deposits (a toxin protein) that accumulate in the brains in those suffering from lack of sleep, and these deposits accumulate over time, killing the surrounding cells. Studies are showing that when we don't get enough sleep, plaque builds up, attacking the brain's deep sleep–generating regions. It creates a cycle where we can't recover from the damage of the sleeplessness.[13] As we age, this cycle becomes more acute. The amount of sleep we need actually becomes more,

[11] Walker, Matthew P. Why We Sleep: Unlocking the Power of Sleep and Dreams. Scribner, an Imprint of Simon & Schuster, Inc., 2018

[12] Mendelsohn, Andrew R., and James W. Larrick. "Sleep facilitates clearance of metabolites from the brain: glymphatic function in aging and neurodegenerative diseases." *Rejuvenation Research* 16.6 (2013): 518-523.

[13] McEwen, Bruce S. "Sleep deprivation as a neurobiologic and physiologic stressor: allostasis and allostatic load." *Metabolism* 55 (2006): S20-S23.

but most older adults are getting less. The loss of deep sleep caused by this hinders our ability to make new memories and restores our capacity for learning. In the case of Aaron, his brain at thirty-seven can recover from sleeplessness, but at sixty, his brain will have a much harder time and Alzheimer's and diseases like it are much more likely. Health has to be more than just today. That gives us our immediate call to action and gets us motivated to find those superpowers, but it is also so important to remember you will want superpowers at sixty, seventy, and beyond. You are sleeping for that brain to be healthy.

Do I Need a Sleep Tracker?

Wearables, like Fitbit, have changed how we interact and measure our health. Apps have continued to put our health in our hands. We can get to a healthful society with health knowledge being with us at all times. But how can we apply those tools to our lives? How do we make longevity part of our daily goals and not just something we worry about later? How can we define success for longevity? In the United States, current life expectancy is 78.69 years, which has dropped slightly due to the opioid crisis. The opioid crisis to me is a screaming call to action. As a society, we need to move away from pharmaceuticals as a quick fix. Chronic pain management with cognitive behavior therapy and mindfulness and other treatments has been shown to be as effective with only positive side effects. You need to shift your focus on health from a one-time, quick fix to a journey of health. That journey will have ups and downs, but if we can own it, we also get to own the benefits of quality of life and longevity.

Susan did not use a tracker to improve her sleep. When Chili-Pad first came out, Fitbit was all about steps. It changed how we think about exercise. But tracking sleep can be hard, and it is a heated debate about how accurate they are. Most have a hard time distinguishing between different stages of sleep. In general, they will tell you if you are awake or asleep. The biggest problem I have with them is their sleep score. Studies have shown that those warm scores can actually make us feel worse about ourselves and our sleep.[14] If they can't tell what stage, you are in and for how long, then they shouldn't comment on quality. Their numbers are a measurement of how much sleep you got compared to the eight-hour time period. They may score you on how much you move during your sleep.

They may score you on your exercise and other health metrics as well. I encourage you to take this evaluation on as part of your self-evaluation. Whether you are pushing yourself too hard or not hard enough is subjective, and an app that tries to score it compared to the whole population is not going to be accurate for you.

If you wear a wrist tracker, it uses an actigraph sensor. If you use a smart phone, your sleep tracker app on the phone uses the accelerometer function to measure your body movement. It also may use sound to detect that movement or other sleep factors such as snoring or sleep apnea. In general, they all make assumptions on your body movement in sleep. While we switch positions during sleep and may be make smaller movements during dreams, we move less when we are asleep versus awake. Some wearable trackers have the capability of measuring your heart rate (HRM). A mattress strip tracker uses ballistocardiographs (BCGs) to measure heart rate and maybe more accurate. I encourage you to listen to your body first because it is the most accurate way to tell if you are sleeping better.

Some people have undergone sleep studies in sleep clinics. In this case, a sleep technician will monitor electrooculography

---

[14] Baron, Kelly Glazer, et al. "Orthosomnia: Are some patients taking the quantified self too far?." *Journal of Clinical Sleep Medicine* 13.02 (2017): 351-354.

(EOG), which measures your eye movement; electrocardiography (ECG), which measures your heart rate; and electroencephalography (EEG), which monitors your brain waves. EEG is the reason polysomnograms, which is the device used for measurements in a sleep lab, are considered the most accurate. In cases involving sleep apnea, specifically, they are needed. But as someone who has a hard time potentially sleeping in my own bed, sleeping in a lab hooked up to machines and wires, while someone watches you might not work for me.

You do not need any sleep tracker to follow my recipe and I highly encourage you to go without to start. But if you get hooked on refining your sleep, I recommend the OURA ring. It accesses the blood volume pulse (BVP) from your finger. It will give you resting heart rate and heart rate variability which will allow you to geek out on your sleep. Studies have shown it to be about 90 percent as accurate as a polysomnogram, but for me it is in my home with me every night and that makes it better.[15]

Health and Longevity versus Age

Dave Asprey, of Bulletproof coffee fame, has plans to die "when he wants," saying that that goal is to live to 180 years. For me it is less about the total years. Maybe it is my physicist notion that time is relative and a poor variable when it comes to measuring age. The universe is measured with entropy not time. Entropy is defined as the amount of disorder or heat in a closed system. You as a human being are a closed system. Your body manages the amount of disorder in it every day. The example of the toxins in your brain, for example: is your body moving to manage the amount of total

---

[15] de Zambotti, Massimiliano, et al. "The sleep of the ring: comparison of the OURA sleep tracker against polysomnography." *Behavioral sleep medicine* 17.2 (2019): 124-136.

entropy in your brain? How does this apply to health? I believe that entropy and disorder are a good indicator of our health. If we think of good health as managing the disorder in our lives, distressing and letting our bodies manage the disorder in our body's numerous systems then we want to sleep to aid in that process. The visual of a peaceful sleeping body is the opposite to disorder.

There are areas, sub pockets of humans, that exemplify this life. They have been coined as blue zones by Dan Buettner.[16] People in these zones have things in common besides having longer-than-average lifespans. They feel like they belong and have a purpose; they are able to destress and make time to walk, sleep, and live. There is a recipe and equation here. How can we take this into our lives? Communities following the "Blue Zone Project" have had huge results in health metrics. This, for me, is proof that focusing on our own state of mind and health will change the outcome of our life and longevity.

Of course, I need to put this into an equation then:

Longevity = (Healthy + Happy) * Sleep

I firmly believe that sleep is the multiplier. Not sleeping has been linked to depression, diabetes, and heart problems. Having a daily schedule that doesn't match your body clock has also been connected to poor mental performance and the ability to make good decisions. Not sleeping lowers your earning potential and crushes productivity. A study from the RAND institute found that "sleep deprivation is linked to lower productivity at work, which results in a significant amount of working days being lost each year. On an annual basis, the U.S. loses an equivalent of around 1.2 million working days due to insufficient sleep. This is followed by

---

[16] Buettner, Dan. "Blue Zone Lessons." *Blue Zones*, 2019, www.bluezones.com/dan-buettner/.

Japan, which loses on average 600,000 working days per year. The UK and Germany both lose just over 200,000 working days. Canada loses around 80,000 working days."

A huge factor in our sleep is our biological clock, our circadian rhythm, or the fancy word for our person rhythm: chronotype. Chronobiology – the science of the biological clock that is governed by a temperature and light-dark cycle – was just recognized in 2017. When the Nobel Prize in Medicine was awarded to three researchers, Jeffrey C. Hall, Michael Rosbash and Michael W. Young, for their discovery of the molecular mechanisms controlling the body's circadian rhythm it validated the importance of your circadian rhythm and its role in your health.

"Workplaces should be making the connection between chronotypes and how we're designed to work," says Amantha Imber, organizational psychologist PhD, CEO of innovation consultancy Inventium, and author of Creating Your Most Productive Workday. In another study, Celine Vetter, at the University of Colorado at Boulder, stated, "You can't put everyone into the same mold, biologically. You want people to be working when they're at peak mental performance."[17] An article in Inc, stated that "80% of employees may work a schedule that doesn't match their natural clocks."[18] Only about 13 percent of people naturally sleep from around midnight to 8:00 a.m.; 56 percent of people would sleep better later and about a third would go to bed earlier. But culturally, we are told to push harder and get there earlier and that those people who work longer hours get better reviews.

---

[17] Imber, Amantha. "Micro productivity: how leaders can make small changes to create huge leaps in performance." *Training & Development* 46.1 (2019): 41.

[18] Zetlin, Minda. "Want More Productive Employees? Match Their Work Schedules to Their Internal Clocks." *Inc.com*, Inc., 7 Jan. 2019, www.inc.com/minda-zetlin/productivity-sleep-chronotypes-internal-clock-night-owls.html.

Chronotypes are more than just early birds and night owls. It is truly a clock that sketches a timeline for the various activities in your day. Matching your day to your clock means more alertness and better cognitive ability, cardiovascular and muscle strength and reaction times, liver function, digestion, and, of course, sleep. Chronotypes have a genetic basis and are linked to your PER3 gene. Your PER3 gene is part of the Period family of genes. A gene is made up of DNA and is part of your heredity framework, which determines everything, in this case, circadian pattern, the primary pacemaker and clock in your brain.[19] The more early bird you are (going to bed around nine o'clock and getting up between five and six) the longer your PER3 genes; the more night owl you are (going to bed around eleven or twelve o'clock and waking up between seven and eight), the shorter those genes. The length of your PER3 gene is also tied to how much sleep you need. Knowing what your chronotype is helps you match your circadian rhythm or biological clock to your day and night.

Are sleep and chronotypes predetermined? It is a bit of genetics – genotype and phenotype. Phenotype is more effected by what you eat and drink or your environmental factors. Picture a flamingo. The bright pink is well known. With a name that derives from the Spanish or Portuguese word meaning "flame-colored," you would naturally assume that it is just a part of them. Though it is their most famous quality, the pink of the flamingo's feathers is not a hereditary or genetic trait. The birds are, in fact, born a dull gray. If it's not a part of their DNA, why do these birds take on shades of pink and red? The bright pink color of flamingos comes from beta

---

[19] Ruiz, Francieli, et al. "PER3 POLYMORPHISMS, MORNINGNESS-EVE-NINGNESS AND DEPRESSION: PRELIMINARY EVIDENCE IN A BRAZIL-IAN FAMILY-BASED COHORT, THE BAEPENDI HEART STUDY." *European Neuropsychopharmacology* 29 (2019): S972.

carotene, a red-orange pigment that's found in the algae, larvae, and brine shrimp that flamingos eat. Suddenly the phrase "You are what you eat" comes to mind. But it points out the difference and the power of looking at phenotype and genotype. Phenotype is a characteristic that comes from our interaction with our environment. Sleep is different, part of both genetics and phenotype. It boils down to knowing who you are and what parts of the sleep mechanism we can influence and which parts we need to respect and honor in our biology. As we dive into our recipe, we will focus further on understanding chronotype further.

Healthy = Diet and Exercise

When you think of being healthy, it is usually about diet and exercise. I am not satisfied with that general look, so I wanted to know how diet compared to exercise as a factor in health. If I am going to spend my time, what should that split be? Miller, WC et al., studied this and came up with "as a rule of thumb, weight-loss is generally 75% diet and 25% exercise." [20] Your best bang for the buck is eating smart, but if you combine diet and exercise then your results are 3.8 times more effective than weight loss alone. I like this because as we get older, the intense daily CrossFit class may not still feel good. But it does tell us that maintaining some level of physical exercise is a big part of that bigger health equation and we can find balance in the fight over which gets more time in our day and thoughts.

Stress?

The next big part of the equation is stress. I recently went on a safari and we walked with two mostly tame female white lions – huge, beau-

---

[20] Goggins, Makayla. "Association of dietary behaviors, macro-nutrients and energy intake with body fat percentage, lean mass, and bone mineral density." (2019).

tiful killers. We as a group walked with their handlers in the South African bush. With us, we had Hadyn, who, at eight, was clearly the youngest in the group. We kept him in the middle of the herd. It was truly a moment where "stick with the herd" took on a whole new meaning. I felt scared; I was not the apex predator. At one point, a gazelle wandered in front of our group and the two lionesses took off. My body surged with adrenaline, cortisol, and a rush of stress outputs. It did what it was supposed to. It prepared my body to have a limb torn off by a lion. It shut down systems like digestion and healing. It increased blood pressure and caused my heart to race. But the lionesses ate the gazelle instead, and my stress abated. When we are in traffic, get in a fight, or get stressed out, our body responds like mine did with the lions. But we are not about to die. We are more productive with a little stress, and we get bursts of cortisol when we workout. But can we relax after the lionesses have left? Can we stop the stress cycle? We need to. Stress is a huge factor in insomnia but also chronic disease, depression, anxiety, and mental illness. For most of us, there are no lions, and we need to create rules and recipes to stop stress and cycle to peaceful in order to balance the equation.

Happy?

Numerous studies have shown that gratitude and relationships counter the loneliness and lack of purpose that destroy our health. Jimmy Carter is ninety-five with good blood pressure and a good diet and gets exercise. He is also focused on his network. There is not an equation for a healthy hermit. We need to belong; we need to feel a sense of purpose. Jimmy Carter still goes to Habit for Humanity and helps build houses for others. He has a high sense of greater purpose in his life. Putting yourself in the position to exercise your happy is crucial. In Radha Agrawal's book, Belong, she talks about getting your daily dose:

Dopamine: "Get stuff done." Have purpose.

Oxytocin: Give hugs, connect, physically share space with other people you care about. Have Sex.

Serotonin: Get outside. Not just on the way to your car. Spend 20 minutes or more.

Endorphins: Workout, get your heart beating. "Sweat. Dance. Laugh."[21]

We will look into these magical brain chemicals later, but these are all a big part of being happy. Dozens of studies have shown that people with healthy relationships are happier, have fewer health problems and live longer.

I end up with a full Longevity equation that looks like:

$$Healthy = 3x\ Diet + Exercise$$

$$Happy = Gratitude - Stress\ (Gratitude\ Summing\ Up$$
$$Mindfulness,\ Spirituality,\ Religion,\ Family,$$
$$and\ Community)$$

$$So,\ Longevity = [(3xdiet + Exercise) + (Gratitude - Stress)]$$
$$X\ Sleep.$$

My father passed away recently. He lived a full life. He was diagnosed with stage four esophageal cancer. He died a little over a month after diagnosis. My approach to death is careful but respectful, I think. Death is something we all have in common. It is a process that allows our bodies to become part of the cycle of life when we are done. Our bodies are the vehicle we use while we are here. I want my body to be happy and highly functional until I am done being here. I don't believe that we can decide the why, but how and

---

[21] Agrawal, Radha. *Belong: Find Your People, Create Your Community, and Live a More Connected Life.* Workman Publishing, 2018.

what quality our life has it the most important piece to me. Sleep is a big part of holding on the best qualities of me.

Kryptonite

When I look at the equation above, it is clear to me sleep makes all the good things in my life better. I want to have that superpower. But the superpower becomes kryptonite when it isn't working. I love the ideal and innocence of superman. He isn't motivated by money or power. I am sentimental about him as a superhero. But I don't think that I am alone.

> *"Superman never made any money*
> *Savin' the world from Solomon Grundy*
> *And sometimes I despair*
> *The world will never see another man like him*
> *Hey Bob, Supe had a straight job*
> *Even though he coulda smashed through*
> *Any bank in the United States*
> *He had the strength, but he would not*
> *Folks said his family were all dead*
> *Planet crumbled, but Superman he forced himself*
> *To carry on, forget Krypton, and keep goin'"*
>
> *— Crash Test Dummies*

The journey you started by reading this book, by challenging your sleep, by facing the emotional baggage that insomnia has left on your doorstep is not easy. To find your superpower of sleep, you will need to humbly respect your body and fight those cultural idioms that say sleep doesn't matter. Yes, there is money and productivity potentially on the side of sleep as the RAND study[22] points out, but it will be for you, your longevity, your purpose and relationships that make this quest possible.

[22] Barnes, Christopher M., and Nathaniel F. Watson. "Why healthy sleep is good for business." *Sleep medicine reviews* (2019).

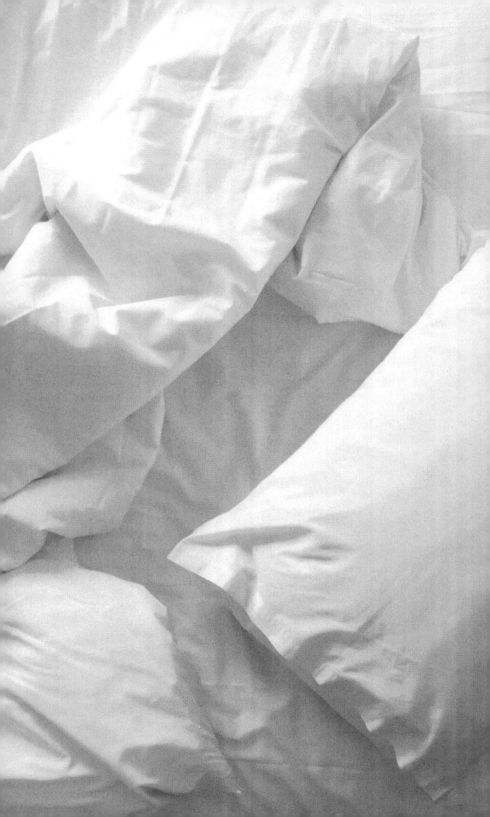

CHAPTER 5

Find Your Triggers

"The things that make me different are the things that make me."
— A.A. Milne —

I hold Pooh Bear in high regard. When the Tao of Pooh and the Te of Piglet came out, they were a meshing of some of my favorite thoughts.

"When you wake up in the morning, Pooh," said Piglet at last, "what's the first thing you say to yourself?"

"What's for breakfast?" said Pooh. "What do you say, Piglet?"

"I say, I wonder what's going to happen exciting today?" said Piglet.

Pooh nodded thoughtfully.

"It's the same thing," he said.

"What's that?" the Unbeliever asked.

"Wisdom from the Western Taoist," I said.

"It sounds like something from Winnie-the-Pooh," he said.

"It is," I said.

"That's not about Taoism," he said.

"Oh, yes it is," I said.

— Benjamin Hoff, *The Tao of Pooh*

Taoism is a Chinese philosophy from the seventh century BC that promotes working in harmony with the circumstances of life.

Most people have heard of yin and yang and the search for balance that is part of Taoism. Taoist understanding changes what others may perceive as negative into something positive. When you discard arrogance, complexity, and a few other things that get in the way, sooner or later you will discover that simple, childlike, and mysterious secret: life is fun. In a recent conversation, someone shared how they hated the word gamification. But I think that this process you are now knee deep in has to be kept fun and not stressful. You will need to understand how habits are formed and changed. But how to organize these recipes will fall into how you organize activities into your life. Maybe it will be in a calendar reminder, maybe with sticky notes, maybe on old-fashioned recipe cards.

Being healthful, mindful, and aware of your triggers will take time to evolve and become integrated into your day. BJ Fogg, a behavioral scientist from Stanford University, recently shared a new emotion. Shine. It is smaller than Proud. But bigger than a smile. It is a bite-sized reward for a bite-sized habit change. I highly encourage you to read his tiny habits book for a deep dive into how tiny habits can work beyond just sleep.[23]

I mentioned the Te of Piglet earlier, and before we jump into habits, it is worth a short pause.

"Without difficulties, life would be like a stream without rocks and curves — about as interesting as concrete. Without problems, there can be no personal growth, no group achievement, no progress of humanity. But what matters about problems is what one does with them."

— Benjamin Hoff, The Te of Piglet —

---

[23] Fogg, B. J. *Tiny Habits: + the Small Changes That Change Everything.* Houghton Mifflin Harcourt, 2020.

I believe Te is essential in how we flow in this river of life and are authentic to ourselves. Te is a part of Taoism focused on the moral code inside of us. From a Taoist perspective, it is natural to look more inward in defining Te but also always factor in how outside influences interplay with you. Sometimes Te is simplified to morality, to do what is right. I am going to require you to think and interpret your results. To use the self-inventory section next to be honest with yourself. To own what will work and what won't work for you. You will have to find harmony and love for yourself. I promise to get back on the ranch now and get practical again.

Self-inventory: I think this was first described and used best in the famous book What Color Is My Parachute? It is an inventory of where you are today and what you want out of this program. By approaching sleep this way, you can respond to the various circumstances that come up in regular life – staying out late, traveling, new pet, new baby, new sleeping partner.

First step is to remember buckets. You are not a single line item. Next we will focus on mindfulness. Mindfulness has been shown to improve decision-making.[24] Nighttime is always full of bad decisions. This process will help you describe and define what you need. What is the minimum viable sleep experience? By visualizing success, you will be able to work more effectively toward the goal. Not just a blanket statement of not wanting to be tired anymore. There are pitfalls to making a white picket fence in your head, I know. But there is power in owning your outcome. When you are facing decisions on whether to follow a recipe and take a break, you will have the perspective to weigh that decision against your goal. Honest dialogue with ourselves starts with information. Life changes will happen; this inventory list may need to be revamped. But the process of self-inventory for sleep

---

[24] Galles, Jacob, et al. "Mindfulness and Decision-Making Style: Predicting Career Thoughts and Vocational Identity." *The Career Development Quarterly* 67.1 (2019): 77-91.

and health is extremely valuable to stand true to yourself. You will not be perfect all of the time. But I am a strong believer in the rubric for life. Measure, test, measure. Let's create your measuring stick.

The first time I did an exercise like this was in a group. Andrea was in that group. She was shocked to find out that some of the habits she took for granted were not good for sleep. She would watch TV every night before bed. She had other great sleep habits, like walks and relaxing, but TV for the last hour was her routine. Because we were working on sleep tips and habits in this inventory, she had it there on the board in that yellow sticky note. It stared at her in that moment, and it became one of the things she decided to give up. It wasn't easy necessarily. She and her husband had shows that they watched, and it was a tough habit to give up. But her time went to reading and journaling instead. Within a week she was pleasantly surprised to find that it had made a difference. She and her husband cuddled and talked about their day after reading and journaling. When they watched TV together, they didn't connect the same way. Journaling and reading serve to soften our defenses and open us up to connect. TV doesn't do that.

Okay if you haven't gotten your notebook, iPad, voice recorder, or whatever you use to write lists (I highly encourage sticky notes to start), take a minute to go get it. I will be right here.

Mental State

This is where you get naked. In your mind, of course. Instead of being an insomniac, you are going to separate chronic problems from your identity to a behavior. You are a person who has experienced, felt, and believed.

Summing up You

I always struggle with this. Perfectionists hate seeing what isn't working in black and white. So put good and bad. At this point,

I like to picture sticky notes. Fill a space. Picture that space in three chunks. Put all the facts about yourself into the bottom third. Keep these simple. I would also encourage those type A people to color code behaviors, thoughts, and emotions differently. These are behaviors like a glass of wine before bed. You may want to include sleep tips you want to try. Like a shower/bath before bed or taking a walk. See the glossary for sleep habits. Thoughts might include, "I want to be a morning person" or "I want to be a more productive person." Emotion examples include "I hate sleep," "I love a warm bed," or "I want more cuddle and love around me." If you aren't sure what category it is, that's fine. Just get it down.

Picture facets of the sleep experience: other people and animals involved and environment, for example. Think of things you do that are positive and negative now. Capture things like "I can't fall asleep" or "I wake up" or "I am tired in the afternoon." This is what you already know about your sleep and yourself. Make a note about how you capture lists, activities, and appointments now. If you were to add a calendar reminder to take a walk every night would it work? If not, what will?

Great, now you should have at least twenty-five things. If you can't get there, dig a little deeper, maybe get a friend to help. You could easily have 100 things here. This inventory has built up over your lifetime. If you need to do this exercise over a few days. Inventory means everything, big or small.

Who Am I?

Realistic

Fact driven

Needs concrete motivation

Self-regulating

Social

People motivated
Needs an accountability partner/buddy system
Human orientated
Loyal
Artistic/makes recipes into their own creation
Wants flow and flexibility
Sensitive
Open-minded
Impulsive
Independent
Supportive

Chances are you are some of all of the above. But you need to take this into consideration in how you will implement this plan. Add those facts to the sticky note board.

What Motivates You?

Leading
Getting things done, crossing things off a list
Help others
Repair, fix, solve problems
Competition
Fame and fortune
Security
Control
Proving other people wrong
Risk/rewards

What Kind of Environment Do I Thrive In?

You can become conditioned to anything you use to fall asleep. Sleep is a habit-based mechanism. It's like the child who conditions herself to fall asleep with a particular toy or blanket.

If she doesn't have it, she won't sleep as well, she says. Is the toy changing her sleep? No, but she associates it with falling asleep.

This conditioning technique is called classical conditioning, or Pavlovian conditioning. Pavlov first noticed that his dogs' rate of salivation extended beyond what would be considered innate response.[25] They salivated when he approached or even heard his footsteps approaching. Stimuli that could be considered neutral became conditioned. In other words, stimuli that had previously been neutral became conditioned because of their repeated association with a natural response.

Why is this important? You need to be thinking about tying natural sleep cues, habits, behaviors, and thoughts into your sleep routine. We will focus more on entraining that to your plan later.

What does my sleep space look like?

I did this exercise as part of writing my book. It was so profound for me that I am going to share it. Some of you will love it and others will find it silly, but it is worthwhile all the same. First, your bedroom is the only room in your home that is named for a piece of furniture. You need to evolve your bedroom into your sleep room. Since sleep involves dreaming, for me this is picturing this space as my ideal dream.

Rivendell is a valley in the fictional world of Middle-earth created by J. R. R. Tolkien. It is magical, full of waterfalls, nature, peace. This is my visual sleep temple. I believe that if I were to somehow be transported there, I would sleep. As you look around your sleeping space, does it imbue an essence of that sleep temple. Are you making this space unique to sleep? If it needs work, add it to the sticky notes.

Temperature

Clearly with a company that makes cooling and heating for other people's beds, this is a big part of my sleep. But it isn't everything – at least not for me. As a farm girl, I feel that messy stuff should go in buckets, and sleep is, well, messy. And since the night breaks nicely into three parts, in my recipe, there are three buckets of sleep. At bedtime, when I climb into bed, I need to be warm and snuggly, but this is obviously different for different people, Todd wants his side to be as cold as possible. Picture a slab of ice. This is first bucket, otherwise called the Bedtime Bucket. The bedtime bucket or first bucket includes a recipe of bedtime habits, including magnesium, tea, reading, blue light limits – well you get the idea. I can go to sleep in ten to fifteen minutes. For me the timing for the bedtime bucket is between nine and ten at night.

The next bucket is your deep-sleep zone. There is REM, light, and deep sleep stages all night, but this time is optimized for deep sleep. Our circadian rhythm is dropping our core body temperature toward the lowest point of the day. This is two degrees cooler than your average core body temperature. My Deep Sleep Bucket starts when I fall asleep until about 3:00 a.m.[26]

Deep sleep helps with recovery[27], filing memories, and that overall feeling of being rested. That sounds perfect. Sign me up. Deep sleep likes it cooler. Your body wants your bed to be thermally neutral to cool or even cold. It is important to think about what your mattress is made of and what kind of blanket you use. If your room temperature is sixty-eight degrees Fahrenheit, but you

---

26 Zhang, Nan, Bin Cao, and Yingxin Zhu. "Effects of pre-sleep thermal environment on human thermal state and sleep quality." *Building and Environment* 148 (2019): 600-608.

27 Doherty, Rónán, et al. "Sleep and nutrition interactions: implications for athletes." Nutrients 11.4 (2019): 822.

have a memory foam bed and thick blankets, your body is going to heat up in that cocoon under your covers. This space also tends to heat up as the night goes along and is at its peak when your core body wants to be two degrees cooler. For me, I need my bed temperature under the covers to be more like room temperature, and Todd needs it to be, you guessed it, as cold as a possible, that slab of ice. MMM finding that right window of cooling and wow. Sleeping in the middle of the night is great. Two hours of deep sleep can change the world. You really want to aim for two hours of deep sleep. Deep sleep tends to diminish with age. By the time most people reach eighty, they are getting little to none. It is the most elusive of sleep stages and getting two hours consistently can be hard. Temperature is the easiest and most consistent way to achieve deep sleep. It is important to remember things like alcohol and stress can make it hard to get deep sleep, so if temperature isn't working, check into minimizing both of those.

The REM sleep bucket begins once your body reaches the lowest temperature in the middle of the night it wants to warm up – picture sleeping outside and the world is warming up as the sun crests the horizon. For me, this is about three o'clock in the morning until I wake up. Czeisler, et al., in 1980 documented that REM sleep stages[28] are most dense in the early morning time. You need to get warmer to get great REM sleep and warmer still to wake up. The third bucket for me was about ten degrees warmer than room temperature. Todd, who loves it cold the rest of the time, also needs his bed temperature a little warmer more like room temperature.

My buckets of sleep have changed my life. You can label these buckets anyway you like, but it is important to know that differ-

---

[28] Dijk, D. J., et al. "sleep deprivation: An unmet public health problem. Washington, DC: Institute of Medicine: National Academies Press. https://doi. org." *Handbook of Sleep Research* (2019): 178.

ent phases of sleep and circadian rhythm want specific timing and temperature for your body. You may have to experiment to find the right temperature and timing for these different buckets, but they form the core of your sleep recipe.

Light

There is a small part of the hypothalamus called the suprachiasmatic nucleus (SCN)[29] that holds the light trigger. Twenty thousand neurons are packed into something the size of a grain of rice. When light hits your eye, the SCN signals your body that it's daytime or nighttime. When you think about your environment, you must respect this little grain of rice. Keep it dark for sleep. It will also be used to stimulate sleep when you mimic the dimming of the day in the evening with your lights.

Sound

Do you need a soundtrack for my program? I love music; I love the poetry of the lyrics. A good song can change my day and thoughts and mood.

Okay so this is absolutely a middle-of-the-night hack. Sounds like pink noise, white noise, ocean waves, and falling rain can be great sleep habits. These popular "sound machine" tracks are another useful tactic that may just help you finally nod off. You may want to experiment with different ones if you haven't already.

There are different colors of sound/noise. And when it comes to sleep, pink is the new black. White noise, brown noise – there are lots of color options. But how are they different? Color of sound

---

[29] Ali, Amira AH, et al. "Connexin30 and Connexin43 show a time-of-day dependent expression in the mouse suprachiasmatic nucleus and modulate rhythmic locomotor activity in the context of chronodisruption." *Cell Communication and Signaling* 17.1 (2019): 61.

can contain all of the frequencies that humans can hear (ranging from 20 hertz to 20,000 hertz. But in general, humans hear pink noise, for example, as more "static."

In a study from 2017, pink noise increased deep sleep and dramatically improved memory in older adults.[30] Pink noise actually helps to facilitate the brain activity associated with deep sleep. While there isn't great research comparing different types of sound and sleep, pink noise maybe worth a try. Whatever works for you is what matters.

Pink, White, Brown?

The high-frequency energy of pink noise is lower than that of white noise. Pink noise contains the same total amount of energy within each octave. Thus, the total energy between 1 kHz and 2 kHz is the same as the energy between 2 kHz and 4 kHz. With white noise, the energy between 1 kHz and 2 kHz is equivalent to just half of the energy between 2 kHz and 4 kHz.

Pink noise is most commonly recommended for sleep treatment.[31] White noise is simpler and contains more high-frequency energy, but some people can find it to be unpleasant. Brown noise is more pleasant but is not generally used for sleep, perhaps because it does not contain as much high-frequency energy as pink and white noise. Brown noise is far easier to tolerate and resembles the deep roar of a waterfall. Brown noise, however, does not stimulate the higher-frequency regions of the auditory system to the same degree.

---

[30] Papalambros, Nelly A., et al. "Acoustic enhancement of sleep slow oscillations and concomitant memory improvement in older adults." *Frontiers in human neuroscience* 11 (2017): 109.

[31] Hilditch, Cassie J., Jillian Dorrian, and Siobhan Banks. "Time to wake up: reactive countermeasures to sleep inertia." *Industrial health* (2016): 2015-0236.

Some suggest the need for caution over using "low-quality" pink noise. "Low-quality" sources include low-quality MP3s, using YouTube for a pink noise source, or using an equalizer.

Pink Noise on YouTube

YouTube is one of the top results for pink noise in a Google search, leading some to use this pink noise for therapy. An analysis of the first ten results for pink noise on YouTube found the following[32]:

- Four out of ten of "pink noise" recordings on YouTube were actually brown noise (much less high-frequency content)
- Two out of ten of "pink noise" recordings on YouTube were neither pink nor brown noise (see the following).
- Four out of ten of "pink noise" recordings on YouTube were actually pink noise
- All but one video had frequencies above 15.5 kHz removed due to YouTube's standard audio compression.

As you can see, you can get detailed on the sounds you listen to, just like finding that perfect song for the mood you are in. If the sound of a babbling brook drives, you up a wall? No worries. Whatever you find relaxing works. Todd is a techno music fan, and for a while as a baby our son Caleb would only fall asleep to MOBY. For me, that would be the last thing that worked. But it has a steady beat, and it worked for him.

Earbuds or no? Comfort and personal preference should be your guide. Some headphones can be in a headband, so they don't have to have the earbuds in their ears, maybe that works for you. I hate anything in my ears, so it is a pain when Todd snores. There's also no hard-and-fast rule regarding volume. But don't worry about being too specific on your sticky notes. You can change the details later.

---

[32] Ziemer, Tim, Nuttawut Nuchprayoon, and Holger Schultheis. "Psychoacoustic Sonification as User Interface for Human-Machine Interaction." *arXiv preprint arXiv:1912.08609* (2019)

High-Level Goals

Who and what do you seek better sleep for? Obviously for you. This is where you take the kernel of you. That piece of your soul that makes you unique and give it purpose. How can you transform that unchangeable piece of you into a mission statement for this process? What do you hope to get from better sleep? In Susan's case, it was productive mornings and being a better mom. For me, it was better health, less stress, and better quality of life. What do you think better sleep will give you? People with a purpose are more positive, are more likely to achieve their goals, and are less likely to fail. A study by Shirley et al. (2018), found that participants had fewer sleep disturbances and more successful outcomes with a higher sense of purpose.[33] More studies into happiness and well-being tied longevity and wellness to happiness and purpose.

To Be Happier?

Happiness and well-being have two general perspectives in philosophy. Hedonic focuses on happiness and defines well-being in terms of gaining pleasure and avoiding pain. In your case, for sleep, this means avoiding sleeplessness. Eudaimonic focuses on purpose and self-realization and defines well-being as a quality in how we function. Our goal for this sleep recipe is to gain both higher functionality and less pain from sleep, as well as more pleasure in your life and relationships when you are rested.

Tracey and Brad provide two examples of how they incorporated this into their goals. Tracey felt exhausted all the time. She felt like she had to take Ambien every night or she would not sleep. She recognized that by giving one month to develop a sleep routine

---

33   Musich, Shirley, et al. "Purpose in life and positive health outcomes among older adults." *Population health management* 21.2 (2018): 139-147.

that she could get off Ambien and sleep better. But Ambien is easier. She had to define a goal that would motivate her past the pain of experimenting for a month to improve her sleep. She had her turning point when she had to care for her dad with Alzheimer's. It is a terrible disease. (My grandfather had it as well.) When she tied the studies of Alzheimer's and sleep deprivation to how she saw her father's life with Alzheimer's, she realized that she had to change. If her sleeplessness would lead to her not knowing her children and future grandchildren, then it had to stop. She finally made the time to commit to a month of creating and sculpting her sleep recipe. Tracey was motivated by the pleasure of future interactions with her family versus the pain of loss from potentially getting Alzheimer's. These are Hedonic goals.

Eudaemonic a moral-based philosophy that focuses on right action as being what gives you well-being. Brad, had a goal more in line with eudaemonic goals. He was angry inside. Lack of sleep and stress led Brad to use alcohol to unwind at night and fall asleep. This behavior caused him to snore, which is bad as well. But the combination of sleep, stress, and alcohol made his so angry all the time that it was destroying his relationship with his family. He had to use introspection to really look at what he was doing to his family. His goal for happiness was about functioning at a level where he didn't need alcohol to unwind and sleep. His sleep recipe was able to eliminate his false sense of need for alcohol, in the same way it helped Tracey eliminate Ambien.

The difference between hedonic and eudaimonic happiness is in what they value. Hedonic assumes that food, shelter, and sex are most important. Eudaimonic is more focused on a sense of belonging and sense of purpose. How you define happiness is important to your sleep recipe because it will help enable you to define why you want to fix your sleep.

Equating well-being with pleasure and happiness goes back to the Greeks. Aristippus taught that the goal of life is to experience the maximum amount of pleasure and that happiness is the totality of one's well-being description. Hobbes argued that happiness lies in the successful pursuit of human pleasure, and DeSade believed that goal of life is sensation and pleasure[34]. Hedonism, as a view of well-being, has many forms; it can be approached from a narrow, bodily pleasure definition and from a broad appetite and self-interested one.

Many philosophers, religious masters, and visionaries from both the East and the West have separated happiness as described by merely pleasure and pain from this idea of well-being. Aristotle, for example, considered hedonic happiness to be a vulgar ideal, making humans slavish followers of desires.[35] He posited, instead, that true happiness is found in the expression of virtue – that is, in doing what is worth doing.

> "between those needs (desires) that are only subjectively felt and whose satisfaction leads to momentary pleasure, and those needs that are rooted in human nature and whose realization is conducive to human growth and produces eudaimonia, i.e., 'well-being.' In other words, the distinction between purely subjectively felt needs and objectively valid needs—part of the former being harmful to human growth and the latter being in accordance with the requirements of human nature." [36]

---

[34] Lloyd, Henry Martyn. *Sade's Philosophical System in its Enlightenment Context*. Springer, 2018.

35 Disabato, David J., et al. "Different types of well-being? A cross-cultural examination of hedonic and eudaimonic well-being." *Psychological assessment* 28.5 (2016): 471.

[36] Compton, William C., and Edward Hoffman. *Positive psychology: The science of happiness and flourishing*. SAGE Publications, 2019.

Eudaemonic and hedonic theories remind us that not all pleasures result in well-being. Going out late on a Friday night with friends is pleasurable but may not result in well-being. It definitely doesn't help sleep health. You have to find the path to better sleep that focuses on future pleasure because there will likely be short-term loss of habits and activities you thought gave you pleasure. Long-term pleasure and health outcomes have to be considered as part of your sleep recipe. Striving for perfect sleep will result in your best potential.

Better Job? More Money?

Can more money buy you happiness? Sleep is tied to productivity, job satisfaction, and earning potential.

Does money make people happy? You probably have an opinion on this. E. Diener & R. Biswas-Diener summarized their research on wealth and subjective wellbeing (SWB) as follows: (a) people in richer nations are happier than people in poorer nations; (b) increases in national wealth within developed nations have not, over recent decades, been associated with increases in SWB; (c) within nations, differences in wealth show only small positive correlations with happiness; (d) increases in personal wealth do not typically result in increased happiness; and (e) people who strongly desire wealth and money are more unhappy than those who do not.[37] I guess it makes sense that more developed nations have both more wealth and higher quality of life so they are happier. The research does seem to show, though, that once you reach a certain point, more money doesn't matter as much. Trends in diet and fitness seem to match this as Americans in the middle class and above

---

[37] Diener, Ed, Richard E. Lucas, and Shigehiro Oishi. "Advances and open questions in the science of subjective well-being." *Collabra. Psychology* 4.1 (2018).

are more focused on their health. Can we increase the awareness on the value of sleep to make it part of our happiness equation? Sleep requires us to make time for meditation and activities that reduce stress.

Focusing on goals other than material wealth are associated with attaining happiness. Diener.

In America, we are a wealthy nation, and we see images of wealth everywhere. Does this feel different for you? I think, culturally and generationally, this can change a lot. But as you look at the list of purposes and motivations, it is important to listen to your inner voice and pick the motivation or purpose that is best for you. It may boil down to fewer bags under your eyes, but there is a strong case that sleep will help you reach your financial and career goals as well. Whatever goals and reasons you have to go through this challenge, make them strong and personal.

Self-Image?

It is okay to note in your self-inventory that you just want to look less tired. It is okay to put down that you hope to find your partner, spouse, or a new friend if you are better rested. You can put down read more, hike more, be more. Sleep gives you all of those, so nothing is wrong here. Big or little, these are no-judgment sticky notes. Just make them yours, and as you read in the sections above, they need to be strong and relevant.

Spirituality? God? How you effect the people around you? Better relationships? Is it mind? Memory? Brain fog? Health? Define a condition you suffer from today and see it healed through sleep. You need to take notes about what is affecting your sleep. Self-inventory works better when you write it down. You may end up with a dozen different motivation and purpose sticky notes. It's okay. There is no such thing as too much or too little detail here.

What Can't I Change?

> Snoring partner or sleep partner dynamics
> Kids
> Pets
> Commute timing
> Work
> Travel
> What Will I Not Do to Help My Sleep?
> Ice bath before bed
> Magnesium oil on my feet
> Teas
> Expensive interventions
> Standing on your head. Go ahead and write it here.

Don't let this list throw you off. It is meant to plant the seed of what we will do for sleep. If you are successful, you may get addicted to this hacking thing and try things you hadn't thought of before. The bucket of interventions is big. Add sleep tips you wanted to try but haven't yet. Maybe something you read somewhere but haven't put it into your routine yet.

Chronotype

A chronotype quiz is in the appendix. There are others online. Take one and add your chronotype to a sticky note. This is important for your planning. You will tie your sleep buckets to the timing from this quiz.

Stuck?

Write down a story or episode from your life that influences some part of the inventory. Write down as many stories as you need to start building a perspective and picture of you and your relationship to sleep.

Write down how you overcame an obstacle in your life. How did you solve a problem you didn't think was solvable before? Give a step-by-step description of how you achieved a goal in your life. Describe your biggest accomplishment next to your biggest failure, how are they the same or different?

Organizing Your Sticky Notes into Buckets, but Not Buckets of Sleep This Time.

First you will need to organize your sticky notes. I want you to move the top five positive changes, thoughts, and behaviors up two levels and the top five negative things into the middle. This is what is stopping success, right here in the middle. Maybe it is something from the Who Am I? section. Are you too relaxed in how you go through your evening? Will you need to account for free flow in your plan? We will focus on reframing these into positive states and stop the destruction. The pretty goals are on top. When you are satisfied with your results, take a picture or write it down. As you accomplish the removal of bad behaviors, thoughts, and emotions, you will see your goals come into focus. And you can come back to this at any time and adjust. But this inventory gives you a solid foundational view of yourself and sleep.

Using the worksheet at the end of the book, you will start to fill in your plan.

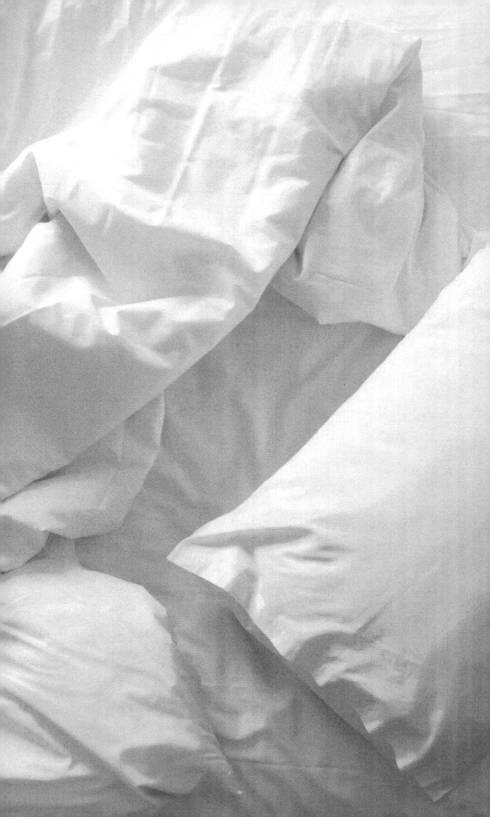

CHAPTER 6

Own Your Blind Spots

"It does not do to leave a live dragon out of your calculations, if you live near him."
— J. R. R. Tolkien, The Hobbit; or, There and Back Again —

We have talked a lot about the why. But you also have to own your why not? I am likely to fail if I have too many things I am working on at once. While writing this book, for example, I would not try to start a new challenge in my life. I would likely fail. If I don't have the support of my family, I will likely fail. You get the picture. I like the idea of blind spots because they can be empowering if you know they are there. If you don't do a shoulder check and check your blind spots when you are driving, then at some point you will fail and crash your car. But regular and timely shoulder checks are prevention.

Now we will tackle those negative stickies from the middle. Our capacity to be successful is limited by who we believe we are and what our genotype and phenotype allow us to express. We need to find the connection between who we are today and our potential self. I am a big advocate of owning weaknesses. We all have them. In order to be a catalyst for change and enable this journey of never-ending self-awareness and improvement, you need to figure out your blind spots. Having insomnia is stressful, and it can cause negative thoughts about sleep. Having negative thoughts about sleep makes it more difficult for insomnia to go away. You are aware of this cycle in your head already probably.

Nathan was and still is a hot sleeper. He runs a successful gym and workout program. All that exercise makes his metabolism rev, and he gets hot at night. His recipe gets him good sleep on a regular basis. But he has a special recipe that clears his head and preps himself for a competition, a talk, or when he needs to be at his best. A marathon runner has a different pattern for his or her routine a week or two before a race. Blind spots and weaknesses are even more important when you need that sleep to count. Knowing these will help you as you build toward your first thirty days of challenge but also when you need to step up your game.

Chronic sleep deprivation and insomnia take a toll not only on your physical health but also on your state of mind. Lack of sleep changes your outlook on life, energy level, motivation and emotions. If you feel depressed, sad, or anxious, likely your lack of sleep is the problem. We need to plan and call out the elephant in the room. Your lack of sleep maybe the biggest hurdle to getting you success with sleep. It is normal in a sleep intervention to feel tired, bored, and irritable or have bad or sad mood swings. It may be testing your relationships already, so focusing on sleep may stress you out about sleep. What are your thoughts about sleep? Does thinking about sleep cause stress? Do you have negative thoughts about insomnia that quickly jump into your mind? You have to push yourself to stop negative thoughts and start positive thinking. This can be challenging.

My company, Chilitechnology, does a lot of work with veterans. I think I see my own depression and sleep mirrored in them. Obviously, our experiences are different, but when you recognize someone else's hurt it creates connection. Andy was in the Special Forces. When I met him, he felt like he was "getting better," but his roommate, also Special Forces was struggling. When you are struggling with depression, self-inventory is especially difficult. Finding someone to sit down with you to work through the physical parts of the inventory from the emotional and thought baggage that is overwhelming you may be necessary. Once we were able to sit down and separate the sleep from the other problems, we were able to make progress. Once Andy had a better handle on his sleep, he was able to also help his roommate. You can't save a drowning person if you can't swim yourself. Settle yourself first, then you will have the sleep superpowers of patience and an organized mind to help others.

Sleep goes hand in hand with mental illness. For example, the National Sleep Foundation found that, "people with insomnia have greater levels of depression and anxiety than those who sleep normally. They are ten times as likely to have clinical depression and seventeen times as likely to have clinical anxiety. The more a person experiences insomnia and the more frequently they wake at night as a result, the higher the chances of developing depression."[38], as stated by the National Sleep Foundation There are lots of expressions, like "everything will look better in the morning" or "just take a night to sleep on it." Deep sleep can be therapeutic to our emotional state. It is logical to assume that not getting it is going to make emotional choices difficult.

For me, I dealt with the grief from the loss of Benjamin and juggled some hefty business pressures when I hit the wall on sleep and needed to find my sleep again. Your sleeplessness makes you

---

[38] "The Complex Relationship Between Sleep, Depression & Anxiety." *National Sleep Foundation*, www.sleepfoundation.org/excessive-sleepiness/health-impact/complex-relationship-between-sleep-depression-anxiety.

vulnerable to slip up in this sleep program. Studies have shown that when we are don't sleep well, we eat approximately 450 more calories a day. Other studies have pointed out that we make poor financial choices when we are tired. Fixing sleep will help all of the other health and career goals, but until you fix this, you need to understand that your current state is a weakness in creating your new habits. New habits require will power. I used a combination of cognitive behavioral therapy (CBT), neurons-linguistic programming (NLP), traditional Chinese medicine (TCM), and thought field theory (TFT). That is a LOT of acronyms. But all of them are designed to break down the patterns of negative behaviors and thoughts. I needed to be fully armed against my blind spots because they popped out everywhere.

I had one moment of how important this was about three years after Benjamin died. I randomly got a call from a woman who just lost her son. I thought I had handled my thoughts and emotions. I thought I was doing okay. But after the brief call – she was just looking to connect with someone else who was surviving this – I was a mess. Everything I had thought I had handled was actually just in a closet. It was exactly how you would imagine a closet with everything crammed in and the door then tightly shut. The call opened that door, and the stuff flew everywhere. I had in fact, not handled the problem. I had only tidied up and stuck it away. I think we all do this. I think Susan had to put the sleep stuff away that was preventing her from sleeping through the night because it didn't seem fixable. When our conscious mind sees something as difficult and sets it aside, even if the rest of our body and mind don't agree. We need to make pathways so when the closet is opened, the negative stuff as a place to go and you can stay on track.

As we build new habit pathways, it is going to be uncomfortable, possibly inconvenient, and require copious amounts of mental energy. As you go through the steps and guides to follow, there will be things that work better for you. It is an ongoing and important part of this book and plan to recognize that you are unique. Find the parts that feel good. This is your teddy bear in the night. Name it, own it, and expect it will get well loved and dirty.

Cognitive Behavioral Therapy (CBT) is a psycho-social intervention. Okay, that makes it sound difficult, scary, and intimidating. But it is, at its simplest, a method of challenging and changing negative thoughts, beliefs, and attitudes. It should help you have some structure to manage that big pile of messy thoughts and emotions that might be preventing you from sleeping. When CBT is applied to insomnia it is referred to as CBTi.

The information included are aspects of CBTi that have been shown by research to be helpful. It is designed to be used by anyone who needs help improving insomnia. But before starting CBTi it is best to consult with a healthcare provider who can provide an initial evaluation to make sure you have insomnia and not a different type of sleep disorder or a different medical or mental health condition. Your provider can also give you specific guidelines. For example, you may need to work through sleep restriction differently than described here if you have bipolar disorder, another sleep disorder besides insomnia, chronic pain, a seizure disorder or a general medical condition. It is also good to use this guide with the support of a healthcare provider.

Let's start with reducing stress by reducing muscle tension. The goal of progressive muscle relaxation is to create a calm body and a calm mind. Dr. Edmund Jacobson in 1908 first outlined the procedure for progressive muscle relaxation in his 1924 paper titled "The Technic of Progressive Relaxation."[39]

---

[39] Jacobson, Edmund. "The technic of progressive relaxation." *The journal of nervous and mental disease* 60.6 (1924): 568-578.

I suggest that you try this out before you need it. This is my own version, so if you find a better way to visualize, go for it. This needs to be a memorized tool, so read it over. Try it and then read it again. Did you miss something? Should it be longer, shorter, include different images?

Lie on your back (I would practice this lying-in bed). Close your eyes.

I start with a picture of a scene in my head. It is a meadow with tall grass on a sunny day with fluffy clouds floating by. I contract all of my muscles and then relax; can I feel them all? Biggest muscle groups to smallest. Relax and contract as you need to. But as you relax, you want to let go of 100 percent. Now can you control this by moving from your toes up and from your head down? Getting this figured out may take time. Can you create a pattern that contracts just your right foot, then right and left, then left calf and right calf with left foot and right foot? Take twenty minutes, play around with it. You can first add tension. For example, wiggle the toes and then relax. Stretch the legs and then relax. Twist the back and then relax. Shrug the shoulders and then relax the shoulders. Bend the head in each direction and then relax the neck. Tighten the jaw and then relax. Wrinkle the forehead and then relax. Close the eyelids tight and then relax. Smile and then relax. Swallow and then relax. If you like you can play music during this time. You can place a warm compress on the muscles you are working to relax. You can breathe deeply while relaxing. You can sense your muscles becoming heavy and sinking into the bed.

Thoughts

This is a complicated one for me. I always seem to have thoughts flying around in my head. I tend to want to worry about things, plan for things. Sometimes these are real and sometimes they are me stressing more than necessary. Sometimes it is only concern or anxiety over whether I will fall asleep. This can quickly turn into a vicious cycle of concerns getting in the way of sleeping, reinforcing the belief that sleep will not happen.

It is important to put these thoughts out of mind and try to turn a thinking mind to a calm mind when it is time to fall asleep. I also use what I affectionately call dream seeding. When I can't fall asleep, I think of a story and place I want to dream about. As a sci-fi junkie it is usually a galaxy far, far away. But sometimes it is a peaceful place like Rivendell from Lord of the Rings. If calming your mind is a big part of your sleep problem, I suggest sticking with one scene and using it as your sleep prompt every night for the next month. Enjoy the story, be your own author, director, and creator for the next month. Don't let the other stuff in. If your mind is full of good and fluffy thoughts, it is hard for the other stuff to find room. Try to keep in mind that you are trying to quiet your flight-or-fight stress response so maybe have it be more drama and less intense action scene. Be the heroine or hero in your dreams. Frame your thoughts as your go to bed to be your own favorite bedtime story.

Most of the time the sleep environment is boring for the rest of the senses: no sounds, no lights, no movement. And so, all of a sudden, it is easier to focus on what is going on in the mind and remain involved with the external world in that way. Go back to your self-inventory and make sure that there are no physical items preventing sleep. For a while I had my workout bike in our bedroom. I had to remove it because it was stressing me out if I couldn't workout. I also have to put a towel over the alarm clocks in hotels because the light is super distracting. This is called stimulus control and impacts wakefulness and sleep. If you lie awake in bed for more than twenty minutes, you have lost this connection of the bed causing sleepiness and falling asleep. In fact, you may have created a new connection for the sleep area to be a stimulus that causes a feeling of being awake. The opposite of what you want.

1. Lie down intending to go to sleep only when you are sleepy.

2. Do not read or watch television in the bedroom.

3. If you find yourself unable to fall asleep, get up and go into another room. Stay up as long as you wish, and then return to the bedroom to sleep.

4. If you still cannot fall asleep, repeat step 3. Do this as often as is necessary throughout the night.

It can be stressful to get out of bed when you want to be sleeping, but the goal is to work hard for a few weeks to months and change your brain connections to be a good sleeper for years. If you are not falling asleep within twenty minutes or you cannot fall back asleep within twenty minutes after waking up in the middle of the night, you need to get out of bed. You have to make a strong connection that the sleeping area is only for sleeping. Don't let your brain connect your sleeping area with being awake.

Sleep restriction is another behavior to help improve insomnia. At its core, sleep restriction is all about reducing the amount of time spent in bed to more closely match the amount of time spent sleeping. What I like about it is it makes sense to not to get frustrated by not sleeping. What I don't want to happen is you use it as an excuse to put off or limit sleep. Sleep restriction does not mean less sleep. It means that you match time in bed to within a half an hour of total sleep. For example, if you get an average of five and a half hours of sleep, I would suggest that you spend no more than six hours in bed. It was first described in 1987 in a research paper by Dr. Spielman, Dr. Saskin, and Dr. Thorpy. In this paper, they showed that sleep restriction improved sleep efficiency from 68.9

percent to 88.3 percent, and the total sleep time improved.[40] This means that before treatment, on average, the sleepers were only sleeping about 70 percent of the total time they were lying in bed. After treatment, on average, the sleepers were sleeping about 90 percent of the total time they were lying in bed. They improved efficiency by 20 percent and slept more total time each night. But keep in mind your chronotype and sleep window; make sure you are in your ideal sleep window.

Important: Do not restrict your total sleep time to less than five hours. If you have any mental or medical health conditions talk to your healthcare provider about guidelines that may be specific to you. Sleep restriction may not be healthy if you have bipolar disorder, another sleep disorder, a seizure disorder, chronic pain, or other health conditions or risk factors.

First, we will learn about sleep efficiency and then apply that to sleep restriction to improve sleep.

What is sleep efficiency? Sleep efficiency is the time you are asleep compared to the amount of time you are in bed. You can calculate this as a percentage by dividing the time you are asleep by the time you are in bed and then multiplying that by 100. If you are using a sleep tracker, you can get the number from there.

Time Asleep / Time in Bed x 100 = % Sleep Efficiency

We will use the same example throughout this explanation on sleep efficiency and sleep restriction. Example:

Bedtime: 10:00 p.m.
Fall Asleep Time: 11:00 p.m. (it took one hour to fall asleep)

---

[40] Spielman, Arthur J., Paul Saskin, and Michael J. Thorpy. "Treatment of chronic insomnia by restriction of time in bed." *Sleep* 10.1 (1987): 45-56.

Awake: 2:00 a.m. to 3:00 a.m. (1 hour of being awake in the middle of the night)
Wake Up: 7:00 a.m. (1 hour of lying awake in bed after waking up)
Out of Bed: 8:00 a.m.

It took one hour to fall asleep, one hour of being awake in the middle of the night and one hour of being awake in the morning before getting out of bed. This is three hours of being in bed but not asleep and 7 hours of actually being asleep. The time asleep is 7 hours. The total time in bed is 10 hours.

The sleep efficiency calculation is: *7 hours (Time Asleep) / 10 hours (Time in Bed) x 100 = 70% (Sleep Efficiency)*

The sleep efficiency can be calculated for each night over the last five nights, added together, and then divided by five to get the average sleep efficiency for five nights.

What should you do about that number? The guidelines for this sleep restriction are from a 1987 paper on treatment of insomnia by the Dr. Spielman, Lauren Caruso, MS, and Dr. Glovinsky.[41] The goal is to get sleep efficiency greater than 85 percent to 90 percent or higher. If your sleep efficiency is greater than 85 percent on average for two weeks, then you do not need to do sleep restriction.

Step 1: Collect information about your personal sleep by recording a sleep diary for two weeks. Calculate the sleep efficiency and total time asleep each night.

Example: In this example it is the same every night – 70 percent sleep efficiency and 7 hours asleep each night.

---

[41] Spielman, Arthur J., Lauren S. Caruso, and Paul B. Glovinsky. "A behavioral perspective on insomnia treatment." *Psychiatric Clinics of North America* 10.4 (1987): 541-553.

Step 2: Set a personal wake-up time based on the needed time to get up for the day. The wake-up time should stay the same every day.

Example: 8:00 a.m. wake up time each day

Step 3: Take an average of the total time in bed from the collected sleep diary information.

Example: Sleep efficiency 70 percent, 7 hours asleep each night

Step 4: Restrict the time in bed to the average time actually asleep. Count back from the set wake-up time to figure out the new bedtime.

Example: Wake up time set at 8 a.m. Restricted to 7 hours in bed each night. Counting back from 8 a.m. that means the new bedtime is 1 a.m.

Step 5: Continue to record sleep diaries. Stay with the restricted time until the sleep efficiency is 90 percent or greater.

Step 6: Once the sleep efficiency is 90 percent or greater increase the time in bed by 15 minutes by setting the bedtime fifteen minutes earlier.

Example: New bedtime 12:45 a.m. instead of 1:00 a.m.

Step 7: Do not change the new sleep schedule for five days. If the sleep efficiency continues to be 90 percent or greater, add back 15 minutes every 5 days until the sleep efficiency drops lower than 90 percent.

Step 8: If sleep efficiency is between 85 percent and 90 percent, do not change the sleep time or total time in bed.

Step 9: If sleep efficiency drops below 85 percent on average for the last 5 days, then decrease the total time in bed by 15 minutes.

After weeks of this hard work, you will have efficient sleep and a set wake-up time and set bedtime. It is important to keep a set wake-up time. This work also helped you experiment and find out what is the best total sleep time for you each night. Maybe you found out that you are well rested and have good sleep efficiency at seven hours per night and you should not be in bed longer than that each night. Maybe you found out that you continued to have high sleep efficiency until you reached nine hours of sleep each night and you need to plan for nine hours of time in bed and asleep each night.

In NLP, we learn that we must be the director of our own thoughts. NLP stands for Neuro Linguistic Programming. When it comes to sleeping, this is super important. NLP can be a powerful tool for improving your sleep patterns. Most people think the "problem" of insomnia is in the evening, the moment they put their head on their pillow. But as we have talked about before, the first bucket of sleep is messy, but it is only a small piece of the sleep puzzle. Our physiological programming shapes how we behave. Sleep has likely become an album you have played over and over again and is now ingrained as part of your thoughts and behaviors. NLP tries to break it down. This is reprogramming. I used to run to Nine inch Nails. I listened to the same tape over and over again (I know, I'm aging myself). But every time I started to play that music my body would respond. It was ready to run before I hit the pavement. Music and other tools need to be part of your toolbox. In the self-inventory spot, was there something that triggers your sleep? Is there thoughts of actions that take away sleep? We need to identify those here. First, you start with the first thirty minutes of your day and work from there.

Here are questions that you should ask yourself:

1. What time do you specifically wake? Is it a simple matter that you wake up too late, and therefore are not going to bed on time?

2. What activities in your day cause you stress and an "unhealthy" adrenaline push? What specifically could you do to change this?

3. What would happen if you changed the way you do these activities?

4. Who is giving you stress? What specifically could you do to change this? What would happen if you stopped seeing this person, or changed the way you perceive them? Is there work needed on a personal evolution level?

5. How much coffee, tea, and/or other caffeinated drinks do you drink? At what time of day? Can something be reduced here or consumed at an earlier time?

6. Do you eat a lot of food late at night? Consider eating earlier.

7. What specifically do you do to relax? And what would happen if you created more relaxing points in your day?

8. Between 4:00 p.m. and the time you go to bed, what activities do you do? Do they involve a lot of electronics, especially close to bedtime?

9. What would happen if you created a "before bed" routine?

10. What specifically do you think about before you go to bed?

The last is an important key. People often can't sleep because they are thinking about things that stress them out. It is amazing how it is outside of conscious awareness that these thoughts don't just happen to a person. When the brain can't help itself, it will randomly start working on its own. The brain needs a little help from its owner. Instead of thinking about things that are unpleasant, or require a lot mental activity, think about things that relax you and/or things that make you happy. Go back to the dream seeding as well.

Other Examples

1. Associate into a moment where you were hugely relaxed. What did you see, hear, and feel?

2. Visualize all of the people you are grateful for and imagine an amazing moment with them. What would you see, hear, and feel?

3. Pretend as if you are going to the most amazing location. Visualize your arrival and what you would do. What would that feel like?

Traditional Chinese medicine, which I mentioned before, was a fascinating experience for me. When I started doing acupuncture, it was because my back was a constant source of pain. But it became so much more than just a way to manage pain. The first book I read on this was The Body Electric by Robert O. Becker. I was hooked. I have always been attracted to energy and how it works. This is where my study of plasma physics came from. Plasma, in this case, is not part of blood but the fourth state of matter. But back to TCM, our bodies are electrical by nature. If you touch a hot stove, you will feel the pain instantly because it is electrically transmitted by your nerves to the brain. Electrical messages are how your body stays informed of what is going on. Without this energy you would not be able to see, hear, feel, taste, or smell. We measure this energy when we read electroencephalograph (EEG), electrical signals in the brain and electrocardiograph (EKG) from our hearts. Our electrical systems are vital to our physical health, which is why medical science uses these measurements to determine brain and heart health. When the energy stops flowing, we die. About 5,000 years ago, the Chinese came up with a system that utilizes the system of energy circuits that run throughout the body to aid in healing.

These energy circuits – or meridians, as they are called – are the centerpiece of Eastern health practices and form the basis for modern-day acupuncture, acupressure, and a wide variety of other healing techniques. It can be hard to acknowledge and put weight in a mechanism that you can't see. Magnetic fields and electricity are not generally seen. We use them every day, but we see only the result, such as a light bulb going on. This energy courses through the body and is invisible to the eye. It cannot be seen without high-tech equipment. By analogy, you do not see the energy flowing through a TV set either. You know it is there, however, by its effects. If you haven't experimented with this before then relax and open your mind.

Energy Meridians

According to traditional Chinese medicine, your chi (or qi) is your energy current that flows through your body via energetic pathways. Those pathways are referred to as meridians, and TCM recognizes twenty of them. Energy meridians come into play here because sleep issues can indicate an imbalance of your chi. Your body's internal clock syncs with different hours of the day, and a different organ (twelve of the energy meridians are associated with a specific organ) works its hardest during the different shifts. It's best if you work with your organs so they can perform energetically efficiently when they're meant to.

How does this work? In TCM, the most common sleep imbalance is related to the liver. Like with Western medicine's circadian rhythm, there are times for different organs, and the liver's time is 1:00 to 3:00 a.m. If you have this imbalance, you would wake during this time and have difficulty falling back to sleep. But balancing your liver goes beyond food; it's also vital to address anger, which is associated with the liver. If you feel irritable, this may be signs of a liver imbalance. The good news is there are tons of methods for leveling out your mind for the sake of your liver – and sleep. Between 11:00 p.m. and 1:00 a.m., the gallbladder is hard at work. The organ is all about digesting, both in a literal sense (by helping to excrete bile and process healthy fats) and also in an emotional one (by processing big decisions and inner resentment). Optimizing gallbladder health, in terms of TCM standards, suggests going to bed by 11:00 p.m. In TCM, the reason the body clock might be off is because you are angry and irritated and causing your liver to be out of balance. To lighten the burden on the stomach, avoid alcohol and caffeine, as well as sweet, pungent, or spicy foods, which are considered yang (heating) foods. Instead, stick to foods that are predominantly yin (cooling). Yin foods tend to be green or pale colored, with a high moisture content. Ingredients such as tofu, cucumber, bananas, watermelon, and green beans fit the bill. Some foods, such as pork and fish, are considered neutral. Another tip is to give yourself an acupressure massage. Located behind the ear is an acupressure point called amnian, which translates to "peaceful sleep" and is used to treat insomnia. It's found between the ear and the base of the skull, where there's a slight depression next to a bone called the mastoid process. Place your finger on this depression and apply pressure in a circling motion to massage it. After circling 100 times, you should feel more relaxed and ready to rest.

Another tip is to massage your lower legs and feet to help encourage the blood to flow away from an overstimulated brain. Better still, dunking your feet in hot water dilates blood vessels in the lower legs, encouraging blood to flow downward. Find a bucket or plastic tub with space for both feet – I have a huge copper one that I got on Amazon – and fill it with hot water. Fresh or powdered ginger is known to reinforce the body's yang energy and adding it to the soak can help those with cold extremities. You can stop the soak once you've started to break out in a slight sweat, which indicates that the body's stagnant energy channels have become unblocked. TCM practitioners believe that when we feel anger or frustration, we're experiencing an outburst of heat in the liver.

Emotional turmoil agitates the body and causes qi to stagnate, which can impair the body's ability to fall asleep. That's why it's important to calm your mind before going to sleep. One way to do this is to practice mindfulness meditation in bed. Focus only on your breath as you inhale and exhale deeply, relinquishing any unpleasant or worrying thoughts. Not convinced? No worries. But I highly encourage you to try acupuncture for sleep and breathing.

Qigong is a traditional breathing workout that manages your breathing to improve your body's health, mobilize its energy and stamina, and improve respiration. Basically, qigong is the art of therapeutic breathing. But if you go to a place online, you can see exercises and flows similar to yoga that will help you with movements – that is, taking a full breath of air into the abdomen. Regrettably, most of us breathe on the shallow side. The key is to breathe deeper. Make it a point to inhale fresh air/qi in through your nostrils all the way down into the abdomen. And don't forget to exhale through the mouth. The abdomen should visibly push outward as you inhale and contract back in when you exhale.

There are also specific breathing exercises to open the spine, which in turn, supports the flow of cerebral spinal fluid. Deep breathing is important in maintaining the body's overall health. It serves to not only properly balance your nervous system but also boost oxygen delivery to vital organs to keep your qi moving. The point is, you have to breathe anyway, so why not do it right?

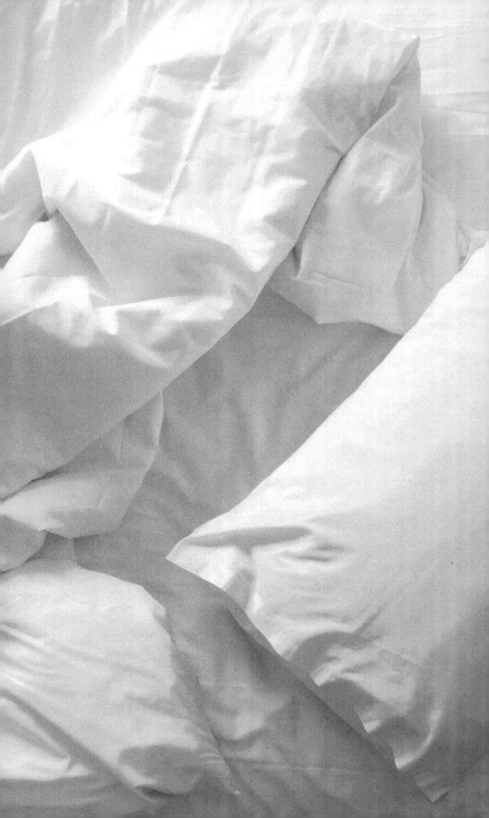

CHAPTER 7

On Your Mark, Get Set, Go

"Motivation is what gets you started, but persistence is the only thing that guarantees your success."
— Edmund Mbiak —

I made the drawing above like a road track because this challenge is a path. You will start feeling sleepless and tired for the first few days or perhaps as long as the first week. But each day you will go into your sleep feeling more confident that you have filled your buckets of sleep with the right things. Each intervention or new ingredient to your recipe needs to anchor to something you already have in your day. New habits floating around without a timing and existing habit to hold on to might get lost. Start small and get those new sleep ingredients to stick to their anchor.

What Causes Behavior Change?

BJ Fogg, of the University of Stanford, calls them tiny habits. He encourages tiny changes as you approach this plan. It's okay to start small and grow in your knowledge of your sleep and knowledge. His book on the Fogg Behavior Model[42] is well worth the read.

---

[42] Fogg, B. J. "Fogg's Behavior Model." (2007).

But we are going to use his idea of attaching our interventions to something you are already doing. Based on the previous picture, we will anchor each intervention to a specific block of time in your day. As you think about when to anchor an activity, you want to keep in mind your mood and new habit tolerance does fluctuate throughout the day.

Morning people should first focus their attention to adding things in the first part of the day. Night owls should add things during lunch time or later. A Cornell University study of over 500 million tweets from 2.4 million users across 84 countries and 2 years found that the content had peaks of positive and negative.[43] It's okay if you feel negative thoughts about this and other things during the day. It's normal. But I believe that when you are empowered to know yourself, you get what has been termed emotional intelligence and can do a better job managing your mood swings. Everyone has them.

If you are a shift worker where your day is flowing differently than this, you will have adjusted these schedules as best as you can. Remember your best time for deep sleep is the middle of the night and after lunch when you core body temperature dips. You will have to get creative, but these twelve steps of your day exist, and I encourage you to make a twenty-four-hour schedule and fit these buckets in where they fit best for you. You will have to pay close attention to creating a chunk of deep sleep time where you are using temperature to cool your body more than an average person might to get deep sleep, but it will get you what you need. I call this sleep density, and even with only six hours of sleep you can feel rested. There is more in Chapter 9 about this.

---

[43] Miller, Greg. "Social scientists wade into the tweet stream." (2011): 1814-1815.

Everyone will be looking at the last chunk of the day. Bedtime. In the spirit of sleep focus, we will start our day looking at the evening as a starting place.

First Bucket of Sleep (Your Sleep Switch)

Pre-Bedtime

I will use a morning person for these examples. Please look in the appendix for the right schedule to match your chronotype. In this pre-bedtime window, your body starts to look for that temperature, light, and stress change. If you are going to take anything to help you sleep, this is the time. Teas and melatonin (this should be a short-term intervention) need time to get into your system. Yoga, qigong, tai chai, and sleep-focused movements are best now. Meditation, reading, journaling, gratitude, and prayer is all timed here. This is a time to dump what keeps you up at night. Make your list of to-dos for tomorrow. Dim your lights is another way to signal to your body it's time to begin winding down. I would set timers on lights to help with this if necessary. Go for a walk, take a bath, read in bed on your ChiliPad if you have one. If you are a TV watcher, try to set up some rules and end your TV viewing to give this time a break from light and stimulation. This is also the best time to cuddle and talk about with your partner. Hugs and touch and, yes, even sex (Todd is smiling) during this time have a fabulous effect on stress reduction and helping us to calm down for sleep. It is tempting to do one more load of laundry but stop and take the time for you.

Bedtime

Again, the 10:00 p.m. time is for example, not set in stone for everyone. You took the circadian rhythm quiz for a reason. Shift this as needed. But don't put off sleep. Russel is a marketing executive. He was a chronic insomniac. Because he was in marketing, he of course describes the fate of sleep for a type A person beautifully. He had "tried" everything. Burned out on sleep tips and sleep inventions, he gave up on sleep. Just like Susan, from the first chapter, he went to bed as late as possible. "No point spending time on something you are going to fail at." Our fear of failing can stop us from the first step toward better sleep. The first morning he slept through the night was amazing. His assistant had his morning coffee waiting like usual. He said he didn't need it. He felt "super." He had his first meeting and all of the meetings that day coffee free. Insomniacs may understand intellectually that they should not fear sleep and put it off. There are no monsters under the bed. We naturally want to put off the things we aren't good at. You will need to be disciplined to stick to your windows even if your habits have led you to stay up and watch the late-night shows or binge watch Netflix.

I love the quote, by Regina Dugan, former director of the Defense Advanced Research Projects Agency, in her TED talk, "What would you attempt if you knew you could not fail?" If you knew today you would not fail at sleep anymore and could have magical sleep, when would your bedtime be? What time to go to sleep would feel the best? Do that time, be that happy sleeper, because yes, you can.

Is your sleep space dark and cave-like? Have you set yourself up for success? Would you tuck in a small child into this space? Is it inviting? Does it feel safe and relaxing? Don't underestimate the power of soft pillows and blankets. I recommend that you get new pillows regularly. In the big picture, fresh pillows and blankets are cheap to replace and can go a long way to changing how we relax into our bed. Don't forget smell. Pillow sprays are another easy add. Lavender is a popular one but find a smell that when you inhale you feel good and want to settle down. This one is more for the girls, but I use an eau d'toilette. This is a light spray, not perfume but it is on my body, so the smell follows me in sleep. In the self-inventory we went into sound. Training yourself to fall asleep to a sound can be a valuable way to bring your sleep space with you when you travel. Having a consistent sleep soundtrack helps me manage the different noises in a hotel when I travel.

Our goal for falling asleep should be ten to fifteen minutes. But giving yourself thirty minutes is okay. Spend your time focusing on what is in your head and what you think about. Take control of your mind. Free-flowing brains are awesome when you are trying to create something but not to sleep. Be mindful and own this time. Stand at the door to your thoughts and let in only what you want. Be the bouncer.

If it is has been more than thirty minutes and you can't fall asleep, get out of bed. It is helpful to have some boring reading, or activity to do. This is where the count sheep thing came from. I don't count sheep, but in a pinch, I will count backward from 100. It takes just enough mental processing to shut down spinning. I have completed this from a 100 and done it again when things have been bad. Stay focused on the numbers entirely, don't let your mind wander. Being able to focus your mind on a single task is a worthwhile endeavor in general because it creates patterns for you to steer your thoughts.

Don't watch TV and try to keep the lights dim. Redo some of your movement and mindfulness activities. Is there an issue keeping you awake? Seed your dreams, think of happy memories and relive them. Your mind at this point wants to follow a path to a happy place, give it one and fill it full of happy thoughts.

Second Bucket of Sleep: Deep Sleep Zone

This is where the magic of sleep happens. From the moment you fall asleep until the middle of the night, your sleep cycles are more heavily focused on deep sleep. [44]Deep sleep is what we need to feel recovered in the morning.[45] If you wake up to use the restroom, you are most likely too hot. During deep sleep your body releases a hormone that stops the urge to pee[46], so if you get up to pee, you did not reach deep sleep. You may also have created a pattern of getting up, so we have to consider that as well; try not to pee just because you are awake, unless you were drinking or have taken something that is a diuretic, try to train yourself not to get up.

Deep sleep wants you to be cool or at least thermally neutral.[47] If you use temperature control, this time should be the coolest of your settings. If you wake up, we have to tackle temperature as the most likely culprit. This is where the patented ChiliPad is perfect, but if you don't want to invest in that, no problem. If your mattress has a lot of foam in it, it may be heating you up as well. Man-made foams are super comfy but those foam bubbles that make it feel great to sink into collect, store, and then reflect heat back at us. Our bodies are ninety-eight degrees Fahrenheit and thirty-seven degrees Celsius on average, and we are looking to drop the core (your inner organs, heart, lungs, liver, etc.) by approximately two degrees. That is not insignificant. Use a light sheet or a blanket that won't trap the heat next to your body. If your room is cool, that can help, but picture that your body is an engine and you are at

---

[44] Yang, Chien-Ming, and Chia-Suo Wu. "The effects of sleep stages and time of night on NREM sleep ERPs." *International journal of psychophysiology* 63.1 (2007): 87-97.

[45] Ohlmann, Kathleen K., et al. "The costs of short sleep." *AAOHN journal* 57.9 (2009): 381-387.

[46] Rubin, Robert T., et al. "Antidiuretic hormone secretion during sleep in adult men." *Progress in brain research* 42 (1975): 121-122.

[47] Burgess, Helen J., Alexandra L. Holmes, and Drew Dawson. "The relationship between slow-wave activity, body temperature, and cardiac activity during nighttime sleep." *Sleep* 24.3 (2001): 343-349.

peak heat: you need to let air flow around you to be cooled from the room. A lot of people sleep naked to stay cooler. I have kids, so that feels a little weird to me; instead, I wear minimal light-weight clothing. If you are waking up hot, another thing to try is keeping a cool, wet washcloth in your fridge. Put it on the back of your neck if you wake up and try to encourage your body to quickly cool down.

Deep sleep is also affected by lingering stress. That is why you need to have built up your oxytocin throughout the day. Hugs give you great deep sleep, and sex can help you get better deep sleep, too. But a hack is to use a weighted blanket for sleep and/or wear socks. These help to release oxytocin as well, and I have to say I am addicted to my weighted blanket.

If you are just awake now and the temperature cues, like the cold washcloths, aren't encouraging you to go back to sleep, give it twenty minutes, using the mental bouncer to keep your thoughts focused on counting or another boring but positive task. If that doesn't work, you need to start with your pre-bedtime list again. Qigong is what worked the best for me. Qigong are movements similar to those in tai chi or yoga but from traditional Chinese medicine. Especially when I hurt, I need to move my body. I printed out a cheat sheet I could use in dim lighting until I got the flow right. I also practiced when it wasn't the middle of the night. There are lots of videos, through Amazon, YouTube, and other online channels.

Your goal is to get up to two hours of deep sleep in this window. For most trackers, this is not accurate, so basically you are looking for improvement of any kind. These days, I use an Oura ring. An Oura ring is a sleep tracker that you wear on your finger. For deep sleep, I feel that it is the most accurate. But if you use the sleep journal/diary in the next chapter, that works too.

Third Bucket of Sleep: REM Sleep Zone

This window should start sometime after two o'clock in the morning. This second half of the night is more focused on REM sleep. [48]Your core body temperature starts to rise. If you use an OOLER or programmable temperature, then this zone should be warmer. Some people can wake up feeling chilly during this zone. Your same toolbox of hacks will work during this time, but if it is close to when you are supposed to or need to get up, just get up. This maybe in your natural window to get up, so don't beat yourself up too much. The timing of this zone may shift as you reset your sleep. My body when it is happy and sleeping well wants to get up around 5:00 to 5:30 but not if I don't sleep. You will need to make the call if this is a "middle of the night" wake up or just an early morning. If it feels middle of the night, go back to your toolbox. If not, then start your day.

I mentioned emotional intelligence earlier. Daniel Goleman's book is worth the read, if you feel like you want to do more work on finding better control and learning to recognize when you are off-kilter. If you are grumpy, own it and fix it. If you are tired, then your brain is impaired as if you are drunk, so treat yourself like a drunk person. Stop the train wreck here. Your day has not begun, and you can steer it. If you are tired, do less, plan a nap or break. Know that the after-lunch slumps may be harder. Plan for the day based on your night. At the same time, if you had a great sleep, workout harder, do more, and make time for the extra fun because you deserve it.

If you feel groggy, then this is the window for caffeine, exercise, mindfulness, or, in my case, a walk and a playlist of happy songs.

---

[48] Marzano, Cristina, et al. "The effects of sleep deprivation in humans: topographical electroencephalogram changes in non-rapid eye movement (NREM) sleep versus REM sleep." *Journal of sleep research* 19.2 (2010): 260-268.

Singing boosts confidence and releases endorphins, giving singers a positive feeling and an energy boost. Singing is a form of mindfulness: so much is going on in your body and mind when you sing that you are fully focused on it. This allows you to "turn off" your stream of consciousness and live completely in the moment, distracting your mind from negative thoughts, focusing on the sound, the action, the breathing, the feeling, and the pleasure of song. Not all people are great singers –myself included – but I love to sing, and it feels great. I always sang hymns to my boys when they were little and up in the middle of the night to help them sleep, and I have done the same for myself on some long, lonely nights.

Wake-Up

We have covered some of this time already. But it is important to continue the thread of governing your thoughts. It is tempting to check the news and social media, reddit, and similar. But before you jump into that, take time to reflect on your night and sleep. What worked, what didn't? In each bucket of sleep, find at least one success and if necessary one thing to work on. If you have tried something for more than three to five nights and it didn't work, try something else. Put on your inner scientist (yes, we all have one). Be curious. This is you, your body, your mind, your health, your life. You are observing and recording you for your own research and knowledge. Don't skimp on this record. You want to make educated decisions when possible. This is the time to record what you have learned and make it actionable. Use a notebook, iPad, app, or however you like to collect thoughts and have it ready by the side of the bed. Sit up turn on the light, not your phone, and do this first. Then take a deep breath, box breath, or do another breathing exercise and open you phone. If you record your thoughts in your phone, try to have the discipline to open the journal first. You are working on your sleep, and it has to be more important than what might have happened on Instagram or Facebook last night.

Morning Routine

You are out of bed. But this is generally a fairly crazy time of your morning, getting off to work, kids to school, starting the day. I am a believer in intermittent fasting. But I also believe in channeling new experience and tests of will power into separate windows. If you are attacking sleep and are in the early stages of owning this sleep thing, don't diet. Don't try a new exercise routine or new thing that may be hard. If your life is stressful, try to pick a window for this sleep program that is less cluttered with big obstacles. This goes for your day. Give yourself a break, reward yourself when things are going well or even just okay. Sleeping more will only help your diet and exercise, so fix that first. But with that out of the way. This is the best window to get twenty minutes of outside time. Can you look at what you do during this time and squeeze that in? Your circadian rhythm is looking for light, temperature, food, and/or water to tell it to wake up. Give it all of these. By flooding your body with wake-up triggers, you are resetting your clock to countdown to sleep.

No appetite? Sometimes if your energy is low, your will not want to eat. It could also have been your habit to not eat when the schedule says but try to have a small morning meal anyway. Even a light bite, like an egg, gives your body the energy it needs to get going. I am not a big breakfast person. I have used a warm tea to start my metabolism instead of food. You are dehydrated when you wake up. At a minimum drink a glass of water. Something warm in your stomach helps you focus. This will make your morning feel more like morning and less like the middle of the night. Aside from getting rid of your funky morning breath, studies have found that peppermint can help increase alertness, so switching to peppermint-flavored toothpaste might be an easy way to stay fresh and focused. For more aromatherapy tricks see the appendix. You can try utilizing pressure points to wake up. The wrist pressure point helps wake you up as well as calm dizzy spells. Measure two to three finger widths from the bottom of your palm, and in the center of your wrist, you should feel a groove. This is usually where your watchstrap wraps around your wrist.

With your right thumb pushed firmly in the groove. Place your right index finger directly behind it on the back of your wrist. Press five times for three to five seconds. If you don't get results from pressure points, do a box breath or breathing exercise to clear your head. It helps combine breath and pressure points.

Morning Productivity Block

This is the best time of the day to change the world, shape new ideas, and conquer the mountains in your day. When I wrote this book I intentional set aside the morning productivity block for writing. According to your body rhythm this will be your most productive time for deep work.

In his book Zenhabits, Leo Babauta talks about big rocks. I am fully in on big rocks. The idea is if you fill buckets with sand and pebbles first, then when you want to add the big rocks, there isn't any room left. His philosophy will double your productivity. I am a big list person. Plan your lists for your week, your weekend, and, of course, your day. Sunday night or Monday morning set your tempo for the week. Have your big rocks front and center each day.

Creative big rocks are better in later afternoon, so double down on the tough stuff. If you can make it work, this is the best time to plan your interventions and set up your routines. This is likely a positive time for your mood as well, so call the relative, friend, or colleague for tough conversations during this time. It gives you lots of time to dump any stress about it as well. Then put in your pebbles and sand but give yourself time for breaks.

Planning for breaks can seem crazy for some schedules, so use restroom breaks if necessary. Back to BJ Fogg, anchor your habits to things you already do. If you are reasonably well hydrated, you probably pee approximately seven times per day. Use them. Guys go in the stall instead and sit. It isn't less manly to take thirty seconds for you. Do a box breath. Eight seconds in (fill your lungs down to your belly), hold for eight seconds, and release for eight seconds, be empty for eight seconds. If you were to check your pulse and HRV you would likely see a change after just one breath. Having a tough morning? Do two. Check your thoughts. Can you turn what may be negative into positive? Can you find a way to separate it from you to a behavior or put a mental space between you and the incident? It is important to limit negative and promote positive. Checking off big rocks. Great. I love lines crossed through items on my list. Back to the dopamine rush. Get your stuff done.

Lunch

What we eat has a huge impact on our mood and body systems. This is where you are best to eat heavy if you are so inclined. You don't have to be on a diet to make good food choices. Fast food and fried things feel awesome when we are tired, but actually the endorphins from getting outside do the same thing. Walk around the block, and you may choose different food for lunch. If you are still dragging, this is where your B vitamins can help as well. I am not a huge fan of the five-hour energies and other energy drinks because most people use them to hide and ignore their sleep problems. But I am also all about a hack, and B vitamins rock for energy. There are other natural energy interventions in the glossary. This is the time to try them. You can also time your lunch break for a workout. Great endorphins come from this, too.

Another trick is napping. As a morning person, napping is not a great idea for me. My genotype also pushes away from naps unless I am sick. Generally, do naps feel good or are they disruptive? Don't nap if it doesn't make sense for you. For everyone else, naps can go two ways: For someone who can't get a window of deep sleep at night, such as a shift worker, longer naps are best (we will cover polyphasic sleep in Chapter 9). But for night owls, like my husband, Todd, short naps can be a lifesaver. Night owls naturally do better with naps. Aim for a twenty minute "power" nap. Caffeine doesn't have any effect on Todd; some people are not affected by caffeine. I will go into tips to keep and tips to throw away in Chapter 12.

If caffeine is for you, then try a caffeinated nap. Drink your coffee or tea and then nap. Of course, you have to be a good napper, because you have to fall asleep quickly. Caffeine takes twenty minutes to hit the adenosine receptors in your brain. When your body feels tired, adenosine is circulating through your body in high amounts. After you fall asleep, adenosine levels begin to drop. Caffeine competes with adenosine for receptors in your brain.[49] While caffeine doesn't decrease adenosine in your body as sleep does, it prevents this substance from being received by your brain.[50] Therefore, you feel less tired. Sleep may enhance the effects of coffee by increasing the availability of receptors for caffeine in your brain.

---

[49] Gracia, Eduard, et al. "Homodimerization of adenosine A1 receptors in brain cortex explains the biphasic effects of caffeine." *Neuropharmacology* 71 (2013): 56-69.

[50] Whitsett, Thomas L., Carl V. Manion, and H. Dix Christensen. "Cardiovascular effects of coffee and caffeine." *The American journal of cardiology* 53.7 (1984): 918-922.

That's why a coffee nap may increase energy levels more than just drinking coffee or just napping.

Another way what you eat, and drink may influence your afternoon is having some spicy food at lunch, which may help cool your body down and help that nap as well. "Eat a hot meal – as in chili hot – because the active ingredient in chili peppers, capsaicin, acts on the same receptors in your mouth and upper digestive tract that detect heat and cause sweating, which of course cools you down,"[51] said Professor Peter McNaughton, a neuroscientist at the University of Cambridge. The thought of a fiery curry or tandoori chicken may make you sweat. The fact that many people living in hot climates, such as in Asia, India, or South America, tend to eat spicy foods rather than "refreshing" foods like melons and frozen treats may actually be based in how our bodies cool. "When you eat this type of food it triggers the central nervous system. This causes an increase in heat in the mouth and will cause the skin temperature to increase resulting in vasodilation – a dilating of the blood vessels – and sweating. This in turn will move the heat away from the body to the skin and then to the air surrounding the body,"[52] says Dr. Christopher Gordon, an expert in human thermoregulation at the University of Sydney. Eating spicy also can charge your energy, but if it's hot out and you want to cool down, opt out of the cool refreshing drink on a hot day; drinking or eating too much of anything extremely cold can cause blood vessels to tighten, making you feel much hotter rather than cooler, so drink hot liquids to cool

---

51 Deutsche Welle. "Does Drinking Hot Drinks on a Scorching Summer's Day Really Cool You down?: DW: 25.07.2013." *DW.COM*, www.dw.com/en/does-drinking-hot-drinks-on-a-scorching-summers-day-really-cool-you-down/a-16974502.

52 Shrivastava, Devashish, Subhash C. Mishra, and Christopher J. Gordon. "Modeling bioheat transfer process and thermoregulatory responses." (2016): 97-97

down with your spicy food. Nerves in our mouths and in our upper digestive tract respond to the heat of the beverage, stimulating the brain to produce more sweat. And as it evaporates, the sweat effectively cools you down. Water evaporates quickly from the skin. And when water evaporates, McNaughton explains, it "cools you down."

But there's a catch.

"Sweating will start, or increase, if the person is already hot," says Gordon. "Whilst people often feel hot during the consumption of the hot drink, they will feel cooler once they are sweating." Sweat glands are distributed across the skins surface. The distribution of sweat glands, Gordon explained, "is greater in areas such as the head and hands and lower leg region. As people sweat, they often feel cooler as they notice the change in skin temperature in the face."

Afternoon Productivity Block

In this block, your core body temperature is dipping. It is craving the afternoon siesta. If your nap fits here instead of a lunch break and napping is for you, go for it. It is also the best alternative timing for deep sleep for those shift workers. Keep in mind, you sleep in 90- to 120-minute cycles and you want to get 2 hours of deep sleep, so if you are going for deep sleep, give yourself a good window. Again, unless you are not able to sleep during the deep sleep window, pay attention to how long you sleep. Polyphasic sleeping can work; however, it is a methodology of sleep habits, and you should try to sleep the same way every day to prevent problems. A one-time four-hour sleep for someone with insomnia, unless they are sick, is not advised.

But since your mind is sleepier and your mood certainly is fluffier and less serious, go ahead and be creative and fluffy if you can.

If you have a must-have-cognitive-fortitude event in this block, it is tempting to reach for sugar during this time, but a (preferably) hot, not caffeine tea will give a similar boost. In America, we tend to want our drinks cold, and as I mentioned earlier, it is tempting.

Try some of those pressure points instead. One of the most commonly known pressure points is located right at your temples on either side of your forehead about the same height as your eyebrows. You may have even found your hands naturally gravitating toward this point when suffering from a headache because not only does this pressure point help wake you up but it also relieves back pain and can help soothe sore heads too. Using your fingertips, stimulate the point by moving in small circular motions. Move clockwise or counterclockwise and do these five times for three to five seconds each. The second pressure point is located at the back of the neck, at the base of the skull. The back of the neck is worth trying as well, it has similar benefits to that of the temple pressure points, but it's easier to activate using the thumbs instead of the fingertips.

Place your thumbs on either side of your spine at the base of your skull, wrapping the rest of your fingers over your head. Massage these points in a circular motion five times, for three to five seconds. Between your thumb and finger, there is a "web" of skin, this pressure point can help relieve aches and pains in the body while helping you to stay awake. Press firmly five times for three to five seconds. To help you locate the exact pressure point, bend the thumb – it should look like a hook – and place the thumb hook between your other thumb and index finger. You should feel a tender spot where your bent thumb ends. Squeeze or apply pressure on the top of your hand in that spot. It should help to get your energy flowing freely and feeling a lot more awake.

Pre-Dinner

Commute, workouts, kids' sports – this time between work and dinner, productivity and home, can easily be filled with stuff. Can you walk during your kids' soccer practice, listen to an audiobook while commuting, or put something else in here even if it is just breathing? There are journaling apps that do voice recordings as well. Maybe you can set your big rocks for the next day. Part of feeling less stressed is recognizing the time you have and feeling good about what you do with your time. This is when I connect with my boys, walk my dog, or sometimes do kid run around, but it feels successful when I know how the day went for my kids. Defining success for each block is important. One exercise I love is from 12 Rules for Life by Jordan Peterson, who uses the example of 100 sick people. At the end of the day, fewer than half will stick with keeping their medication without supervision. But ask those same people to be responsible for someone else taking the medication and they will insist that the protocol is followed. We need to treat ourselves like someone we are responsible for helping.

Dinner

Yes, alcohol makes you feel sleepy and a glass of wine with dinner can be just fine. But it makes it harder to stay asleep because it can make you have to pee. It can make you feel groggy in the morning because it can be terrible for deep sleep. If you can't resist, stick to one drink and have it with dinner, or at least two to three hours before bedtime or try to take certain nights each week off. Vitamin and mineral deficiencies can have huge impact on sleep. See Chapter 9 for more on what to look for and why.

Dinner is the time to connect, to break bread. In our modern world, it is hard to always have a family dinner, but my family does try for one at least once a week. We use an exercise that the boys learned at camp. What was my highlight? What am I grateful for? And what was my daily good? Sometimes having this as a prompt to get everyone to talk helps with connection. Is also helps drive us as family to think and do things we can talk about at dinner. A daily good can be as simple as picking up a piece of trash to helping someone feel better to going above and beyond for something or someone. Make dinner more than just food. This has been a focal point of the human herd connections since forever. We don't need to be on electronics (Super Bowl Sunday is an exception in our house); we need to focus on each other. Don't have people to connect with? Sharing space even in a restaurant can help. I like that when I am traveling for sure.

Try to eat earlier, especially for morning people. A big dinner can make you sleepy but prolongs the digestion process, which interferes with a good night's sleep. It's best to eat your biggest meal at lunch and have a light evening meal of 500 calories or fewer. Include some chicken, extra-lean meat, or fish at dinner to help curb middle-of-the-night snack attacks.

Spicy foods can contribute to sleep problems: Dishes seasoned with garlic, chilies, cayenne, or other hot spices can cause nagging heartburn or indigestion. Avoid spicy foods at dinner. Gas-forming foods and hurried eating also cause abdominal discomfort, which in turn interferes with sound sleep. Limit your intake of gas-forming foods to the morning hours, and thoroughly chew food to avoid gulping air.

Evening

Flop. I can hear one of the boys plopping down on the couch. Christopher Chabris and Daniel Simons, in their book Invisible Gorilla, do an amazing experiment. You can google it and watch the video. Participants in the study are asked to watch a video and count the passes between people in white shirts and people in black shirts. Sounds easy. In the middle of the video, unknown to the participants, a gorilla walks in, faces the camera and walks out. You would all think we would see it, but at least half of the participants did not. It has become a well-known psychology experiment. When you watch TV and zone out, you miss the gorillas in your life. We don't connect and see our environment, and we can miss out on family time. Our minds may tell us we are present, but we are not being present with our kids and family. I love family cuddle-on-the-couch-and-watch-a-movie time. But try to change it up. Don't let your evenings become so focused on TV that you lose your chance to connect. If we don't connect during this time block, it will hurt us emotionally and make it harder to relax and unwind pre-bedtime.

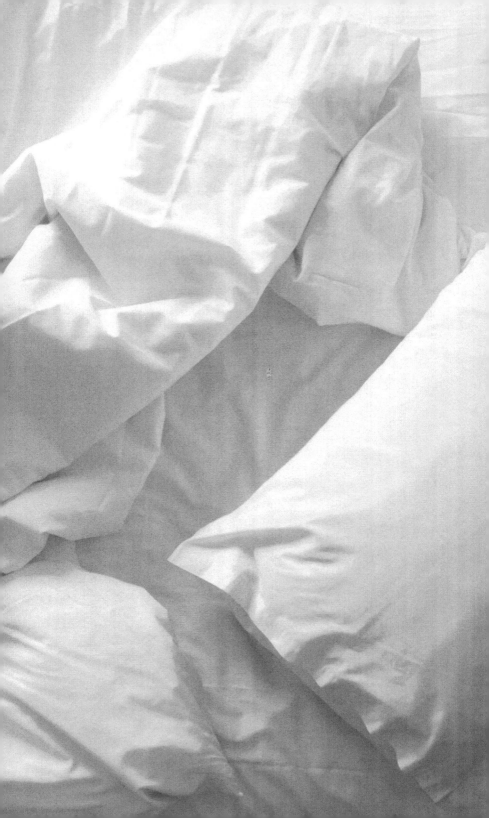

CHAPTER 8

Reflection Is the Key to Success

"Success is not final; failure is not fatal: it is the courage to continue that counts."
— *Winston S. Churchill*

We all fail sometimes. I feel like I fail a lot, but they are only true failures if we don't learn from them. You have failed at sleep until now, and you will fail in the future. But I believe that the way to break the cycle of consistent insomnia is to reflect often and with as much detail as possible. Above is a page of a survival journal. It takes a stab at what you might want to include in yours. Your will-power, your mood will shift during the day and you need a guide to keep it together. Use your journal first thing in the morning to document and track your sleep. You want to target adding each new intervention with the plan to try it at least four days. Test, do, retest – that is the focus of this chapter.

I recommend creating a diary or journal for this sleep challenge and maybe beyond. Todd likes to use a journal app so he can dictate to it while he drives in the morning. I am more old-fashioned and like a book; writing with a pen still feels better. Things to include are:

1. Sleep highlights: the good, the bad, the ugly, and successes too.
   A. If it is just a happy or frowny face, that works!

    B. You may want to include the times you might have woken up.

    C. Write down what worked from the bedtime bucket from the night before.

    D. Just track rested or not if nothing else.

2. Big rocks, to-do list.

    A. Keep stress out of sleep, write it down.

    B. Remember crossing things off your list gives you a natural high!

    C. Big rocks versus sand: organize your day to fill it with what matters most.

3. Take three thoughts of gratitude, strength, and inspiration into your day.

    A. We all need to have our reasons for the hard work in front of us.

    B. It will help you to be prepared for the stress with an armor of good.

    C. If your head is filled with good there isn't room for bad or ugly thoughts.

4. Magic tool of the day: Breath!

    A. It can change but take a breathing exercise, dance move, favorite song into your day.

    B. The clothes make the man: Tough days require better outfits. If it is going to be a tough day, put on something new, colorful, or whatever feels good to be your armor.

5. Magic moment.

    A. How will you honor your success today?

    B. What little treat will you give yourself if you get your big rocks done?

C. What will be a little reward for the first great night of sleep?

D. What is the medium reward for your first week of great sleep?

E. What is the wow reward for nailing your recipe for sleep?

6. Daily good.

A. Spread the love! Find a way to give back; you will be amazed at how finding a way to reach out, even just with an extra hug will make you feel amazing. Don't let more than one day go by.

7. Gratitude.

A. There will always be someone who has it worse than you. Find five things to be grateful for each day.

But reflection and introspection needed for this are more than just tracking your sleep or crossing off your to-do list. Human beings have survived by constantly observing and analyzing. Introspection involves examining one's own thoughts, feelings, and sensations in order to gain insight. But slowing down and taking a breather from our crazy lives isn't always the easiest thing to do. In a society fixated on fast-paced environments and a "go, go, go" mentality, it's difficult to find the time to sit down and reflect. However, setting aside a small portion of your day for self-examination can be a lot more helpful than you might expect. Setting this as a long-term habit will help in other areas of your life as well.

In our case, we look for negative patterns. Maybe you put off sleep or do things that hurt your sleep, convincing yourself that it doesn't matter much. Introspection allows you to recognize these patterns and how and why they have a detrimental effect on your emotions and outlook. The first step is recognition but eventually you can consider alternate approaches to these situations and eventually, migrate away from the stressors altogether. When we don't have an overall goal in mind, our tasks seem meaningless and possibly frustrating. It's important to have a clear vision of where you want to see yourself in the future. This is why you need to outline weekly and monthly goals for sleep. Be reasonable. If you wake up every night, then you want to focus on that, and if we can help other things along the way, then great. If it is falling sleep, that first bucket of sleep can be hard to get a breakthrough. Aim small on your goals and measure even small successes. Try falling asleep 50 percent faster as a first step. Don't forget to continually remind yourself of what you hope to ultimately accomplish: good, consistent sleep. This process will result in a more positive attitude toward your sleep tasks and possibly the extra work it takes to push toward this goal.

Wild Puppies and Hypnagogic Sleep

Your mind is a powerful thing. We have looked at how sleep is naturally managed subconsciously, but that spinning brain needs to be told to stop. Margaret had to spend a lot of time in this place. I confess I struggle with a spinning mind as well. She had a lot of problems in her home and work life to solve. For her, the story of Thomas Edison was helpful. Inventors have notoriously busy brains. Edison was no exception. But instead of spinning on a problem all night, he found a way to limit the problem window. There is a special part of sleep devoted to problem solving. It is called hypnagogic sleep and is a fabulously fascinating aspect of sleep. I was fully introduced to it at a MIT Media Lab workshop on dream engineering. In the moments when you first fall asleep, your mind lets go of all physical parameters. I like to imagine this is like the scene in matrix where Neo (Keanu Reeves) is learning to jump between buildings. He had to let go on the laws of physics and gravity because they weren't real. This is hypnagogia, your brain untethered and free to spin. But if this happens every night, why aren't we all inventors? Edison and many other visionaries and creative types hack hypnagogia. Edison would lie on his workbench holding two steel balls in his hands, thinking about a problem he needed to solve; he would then take a nap. As you transition from hypnagogia to light sleep, your body relaxes. In the case of Edison, he released his hold and the steel balls hit the floor. He woke up with a fresh view on his current problem. Margaret had to set aside time to let her mind spin on a problem. She tried hypnagogic naps. She tried lucid dreaming, a state of semiconscious dreaming where you control your dream. She found ways to use sleep to help but not let those problems run free through her sleep. Problems are like puppies and can wreak havoc in their wake. Put them in their kennel and enjoy interacting with them on your terms.

Sleep Environment

An infuriating dog barks and keeps you awake, you have a stressful day, a torrential downpour on the way home delays your commute and your whole schedule falls apart – you get the idea. No matter how many times we've been told not to stress about what we can't change, we do it anyway. It's difficult to realize we don't always have total control of the outcome, and sometimes, we have no choice but to adapt to what we are left with. We need to focus our energy toward things we can change. You have likely been struggling with this for a while, you may have put some mental blocks in place, and they may block the chance of changing things for the better. By becoming more self-aware, you will have a better understanding of what you truly want from this program. Naturally, fixing sleep will involve making changes, whether they're significant or menial. Of course, nobody likes to change. It's uncomfortable and scary, and we seek comfort in what we know. However, this is why it is critical to ask ourselves, is it worth it take as little as five minutes out of our day to reflect in exchange for an increase of success? Keep positive and continue with your plan to switch things around and keep experimenting. Use the list of interventions and tips at the end of this book, and at least weekly review and change or add things to your daily plan. Your introspection goal is to measure how you feel about your sleep. Even a happy, neutral, or sad face will work. Use this as a chance to also track your mood, thoughts, and when and how tired you feel throughout the day. Keep in mind with this program and all tracking that one night is not enough time to know if something is working.

Should I Use a Sleep Tracker?

If you use a sleep tracker, then you can keep track of it there as well. Sleep trackers are wearable devices built to track data about our health, fitness, and, of course, sleep and then serve those numbers back to us with scores, graphs, and ratings. They are fairly popular, from high-end running watches from Garmin to simple and affordable activity trackers from companies like Fitbit.

"Nearly 22 percent of US adults use a wearable sleep-tracking device, and about half of the nation's population would consider buying one."[53] But even though sleep trackers have become increasingly popular in recent years, many health experts think they're kind of, well, bogus. Not only are the tools fairly inaccurate, but they also don't offer a deep, comprehensive look at our sleep patterns. "The common use of commercially available sleep trackers by the general public should be done so with a clear understanding

---

[53] Ries, Julia. "FYI, Your Sleep Tracker Is Pretty Useless." HuffPost, *HuffPost*, 18 July 2019, www.huffpost.com/entry/do-sleep-trackers-work-app_l_5d2e7c5be4b085eda5 a38aa9.

that these are limited tools that at best can tell you a bit more about your sleep duration and sleep timing," said Dr. Jeffrey Durmer, a sleep medicine physician and chief medical officer of the sleep health company Fusion Health. In an intervention study called SHIP (Study of a Health Intervention Programme) targeting personnel at a correctional institution in Sweden, the results concerning actigraphy sleep measures (which most sleep trackers measure) suggest that data from at least two nights are recommended when assessing sleep percent and at least five nights when assessing sleep efficiency.[54] For actigraphy-measured total sleep time, more than seven nights are needed. At least six nights of measurements are required for a reliable measure of self-reported sleep. Fewer nights (days) are required if measurements include only weeknights. Overall, there was a low correlation between the investigated actigraphy sleep parameters and subjective sleep quality, suggesting that the two methods of measurement capture different dimensions of sleep.

John was an avid user of his Garmin. At seventy-six, he needed deep sleep specifically. He wore his Garmin every night, and it told him he was getting 40 percent deep sleep. Unfortunately, when we had John wear another tracker, his data was completely different, and the patterns went away. The truth is neither tracker turned out to be accurate for deep sleep. This is not unusual. There is a reason that researchers only want to use polysomnographic information. Consumer-grade trackers have a bad reputation. John still loved his Garmin, and he was happy with it despite its lack of accuracy for deep sleep. Instead of having him go crazy with different tracking, we had him look at the data for trends instead of individual met-

---

[54] Aili, Katarina, et al. "Reliability of actigraphy and subjective sleep measurements in adults: the design of sleep assessments." *Journal of Clinical Sleep Medicine* 13.01 (2017): 39-47.

rics. If we were working on his deep sleep and we were looking for improvement, then month to month if deep sleep went from 40 percent to 50 percent, then we made the assumption that it was better.

How Do Sleep Trackers Work?

Sleep trackers typically measure how long you're sleeping based on your movement throughout the night. The basic methodology behind the tool is that when you're awake, you move more, and when you're asleep, you're still. This might be true, generally, but it isn't always the case, said Richard Shane, a behavioral sleep therapist and developer of the Sleep Easy method. "Somebody could be, let's say, a serious insomniac and they have trained themselves to lay still when they're not sleeping, and the activity monitor or motion sensor will record that as being asleep,"[55] Shane said. "Likewise, somebody could be sleeping but restless in their sleep, and their device might measure that as being awake." Consequently, some trackers don't get a scientific look at how long you've been asleep. In certain cases, people who may be zonked out might assume they're missing out on z's based on false data. Some people even getting sleeping tracking while watching TV.

Mapping out your brain waves is the best way to monitor what stage of sleep you're in (like REM sleep, for example) and determine if you may have a sleep disorder. There are some headbands that might be more accurate because of how they measure brain waves. Often times the insights that sleep trackers provide – such as a report saying you got "light sleep" – aren't considered to be clinical or medically sound definitions. Rather, this is more or less the

---

[55] "Dr. Richard Shane, Ph.D. Founder of Sleep Easily Announces Groundbreaking Sleep Therapy." *New West Physicians,* 11 Oct. 2016, www.nwphysicians.com/dr-richard-shane-ph-d-founder-of-sleep-easily-announces-groundbreaking-sleep-therapy/.

company's way of interpreting and making sense of your sleep data. Additionally, most trackers also don't share the reasons behind your sleep patterns or potential steps you can take to improve your sleep. If you do decide to use a sleep tracker, understand that you're getting a picture of your sleep and not a 100 percent accurate view.

Why Should I Use a Tracker Then?

That said, sleep trackers can give you some useful information to work with, according to Johns Hopkins Medicine.[56] Sleep trackers can help you recognize patterns in your sleep and adjust certain habits. For example, if you feel sluggish when you go to bed later, try shifting your bedtime to an hour or two earlier. And if you notice that you sleep more soundly after a workout, make a point to exercise more.[57]

While the trackers can't replace formal testing, they may help your doctor determine if it may be time for you to undergo further examination or see a sleep specialist[58], according to the Cleveland Clinic.

Leading the way are traditional wearable providers like Oura, Polar, Nokia/Withings, and Fitbit, all of which have sleep tracking in their devices. However, some people are fine with how they feel during the day but wearing a fitness band at night is often uncomfortable. There is also a group of noncontact options from sleep specialists ResMed, Beddit, and Emfit. Beddit and Emfit are both basically a strap that looks and feels kind of like a leather strap that

---

[56] "Do Sleep Trackers Really Work?" *Johns Hopkins Medicine,* www.hopkinsmedicine.org/health/wellness-and-prevention/do-sleep-trackers-really-work.

[57] Zhao, Zhengqing, Xiangxiang Zhao, and Sigrid C. Veasey. "Neural consequences of chronic short sleep: reversible or lasting?." *Frontiers in neurology* 8 (2017): 235.

[58] Medic, Goran, Micheline Wille, and Michiel EH Hemels. "Short-and long-term health consequences of sleep disruption." *Nature and science of sleep* 9 (2017): 151.

sits on top of your mattress, beneath the sheets. It is nice not to wear anything, but it is a strap that you sleep on with just the sheet between you. If you don't like the idea of putting a gadget in your bed or wearing one on your wrist, it might be time for you to try a smart ring instead. The Oura ring is an activity, wellness, and sleep tracking device rolled into one tiny, slim package that's about the size of a standard wedding band. Although it can track your activity, the Oura ring is focused on wellness and particularly sleep. It provides you with a simple sleep score each day, but you can delve deeper into your stats to find out all kinds of information about the quality of your rest, from your resting heart rate to how much you moved, all presented on a series of bar charts and graphs. You do get a detailed breakdown of the quality and quantity of sleep, heart rate data, and breaths per minute. It's crack for sleep and data nerds. And I have to admit I am in love with mine.

There are also what seem like a zillion sleep apps out there. Sleep Cycle is one of the better ones, but it still is mostly about tracking. Its best feature is its smart alarm, which "listens" for the right time in your sleep to wake you up and gives a window for your alarm to wake you up. I will be launching EEP in 2020. It will be an app that matches this program and puts all of the interventions in your smart phone. Stay tuned.

Final Thoughts on Sleep Tracking

My advice to people is trust your body more than a device. If you wake up and you feel that your tracker matches how you feel most of the time, then great. I would recommend recording both your tracker score and your "feelings" or subjective reflections as well. Pay attention to what helps you sleep better, by taking note of how you feel. If you want to get into the details of your sleep patterns, go see a sleep doctor. They can conduct a polysomnography, or a medical sleep test, to get a thorough look at the various factors that may be affecting your sleep each night. It is not an easy sleep space though. You are hooked up to wires, and a technician then monitors your brain waves and detects your sleep state. If you snore and think you might have sleep apnea, then this is what you need to do.

If you are not sleeping well and would like to improve your sleep, a tracker is not going to provide you with a solution; it is an only account of what happened during the night. The complexity of our sleep and circadian rhythms requires us to create a plan, including specific and personal medical, well-being, and psychological inputs in order to help you improve your sleep. Knowing whether you had a "good" or "bad" night of sleep is useless, as those terms are based on objective measures that have little bearing on how you feel in the morning. "Unfortunately, we have shown (after analyzing sleep from nearly 5000 individuals) that objective measures tell us little about subjective sleep,"[59] says Dr. Jamie Zeitzer, assistant professor at Stanford University in the Department of Psychiatry and Behavioral Sciences and the Centre for Sleep Sciences and Medicine, about the role technology can play in helping us to get a better night's sleep. "We are often unaware of the actual causes of poor sleep at night. The hope is that sleep monitoring tech will allow us to track the variety of behaviors and environmental factors that could contribute to poor sleep." For instance, a recent study suggested that some people felt more tired throughout the day based on what their sleep tracker told them – not how they actually slept.

My biggest concern about tracking your sleep with tech, is that you manage how that tech might interfere with your sleep and use

---

[59] Caddy, Becca. "Will Better Technology Solve Our Sleep Sorrows?" *TechRadar*, TechRadar, 7 Oct. 2017, www.techradar.com/news/will-better-technology-solve-our-sleep-sorrows.

the data as just that – data. Trust your body and feelings more. Use trackers to confirm what you should already know, and the information is actionable and empowering. Don't let it get you upset or depressed or shake you from your plan. You've got this.

CHAPTER 9

The Powerful Armor of Information

"Sometimes I lie awake at night, and ask, 'Where have I gone wrong?' Then a voice says to me, 'This is going to take more than one night.'"
— Charles M. Schulz —

You follow the rules: drink a tea went to bed on time and – nothing. Sleep stalls out. Your thoughts are still flying things you didn't do today, the fight with your partner, your kid's science fair project due next week. If this happens to you, you are not alone. Stress, anxiety, and runaway thoughts are big culprits in losing sleep. I have outlined some interventions before, but this chapter gives a little more context. There are many more in the tips and tricks appendix, and sleep terms in the glossary, but this will represent the equivalent of googling sleep online and getting twenty top tips, but I will explain how they work and why because without that, it may not make sense when only half, or maybe fewer, actually work for you. I think what is missing in sleep is this path to use and the context in how to use it.

Ty, my oldest son, broke us in as parents. He didn't sleep through the night until he was in kindergarten. Lots of people have the babies who miraculously sleep through the night almost immediately, but I was not blessed that way. But what Ty did give to me was the power of information. Because he didn't sleep, refused to potty train, could escape any room, and didn't talk until he was four, I had to become a better parent. I had to read every parenting book to try to find a solution. Mary Sheedy Kurcinka's Raising Your Spirited Child was the first thing I read that seemed to "get" my life with Ty. The power of that information was more than just the tips and tricks to help me as Ty's parent, it was the knowledge that I wasn't alone with this problem. Everyone else's kid on the playground was "doing the right thing, at the right time." I felt like a failure as a mom. I have shared this book and many of the parenting books I used to cope and grow with Ty with other struggling parents. Knowledge and information are more than the steps they give you. They are an armor against the fear and anxiety of not being good at something or not standing up to your or other people's expectations. Let the knowledge of sleep set you free to be who you are. Ty is a grown up now, and he is still just as amazing and special as he was as a baby and toddler. I still, as a parent, get sucked into the drama of why my kids are not the same as everyone else, and I have to remind myself that I won't want them to be. Each is special and brings his unique purpose and gifts. Your sleep is a child to be nurtured. Don't worry that he isn't talking or potty trained when other kids are. Just enjoy loving it for being yours. We cannot discount what makes us special is a gift, even the parts that frustrate us for not being the same as everyone else.

Meditation

Meditation is absolutely one of those tips that you read about and wonder how it works or how to apply it to helping you sleep. I felt that even after downloading Headspace, I did not know what it was all about. I at least had someone in my ear telling me how to do it. But my research told me it works. Great. But how can it help me sleep? Meditation helps with stress[60], but how do I take that swirl of thoughts at night and translate that to meditation? I put on a recording of meditation and it encourages me to clear my head, but my head doesn't always want to listen. I had to make meditation my own before it worked for me. I had to feel the results and be able to use the why for me. Blindly playing the app, it took me several sessions to start to change my thoughts. I actually found more success in combining activity like yoga and qigong with meditation to start. My mind races like a full-speed race car – zero to sixty in under three seconds, and it doesn't want to stop on a dime. Meditation is a training exercise to enable you to control your thoughts and body. You learn to differentiate between a helpful thought and a destructive one. Meditation also rewires your brain, strengthening neural pathways that calm your nervous system.

Deana was not someone who had ever heard of meditation – well, other than an image of a Buddhist monk and lots of silence. It was intimidating for her. At sixty-three, she wasn't about to sit cross legged on the floor and chant. It didn't matter what the results might be. She started mediating in her bed lying down flat. She fell in love with yoga nidra to start and now takes yoga classes regularly and has four qigong exercises she does before bed. You don't have to jump into the deep end with this meditation thing. Start small; peaceful thoughts can be addicting, and you will soon be listening to your body enough that you can move on to bigger challenges.

I like both qigong and yoga nidra. But yoga nidra is a fabulous place to start meditation.[61] In Hindi, it actually means sleep

---

[60] Greeson, Jeffrey M., et al. "Mindfulness meditation targets transdiagnostic symptoms implicated in stress-related disorders: Understanding relationships between changes in mindfulness, sleep quality, and physical symptoms." *Evidence-Based Complementary and Alternative Medicine* 2018 (2018).

[61] Datta, Karuna, Manjari Tripathi, and Hruda Nanda Mallick. "Yoga Nidra: An innovative approach for management of chronic insomnia-A case report." *Sleep Science and Practice* 1.1 (2017): 7.

yoga. It isn't just trying to lie still and be peaceful to calm your thoughts. But it starts with exactly that. A lot of meditation experts say that this style of yoga can equal deep sleep because it offers such deep recovery. While more conclusive studies are necessary to understand precisely why this is so, researchers believe it's related to the brainwave changes you undergo during yoga nidra. This isn't like the yoga class at the Y. This yoga is basically dynamic sleep. It is looking for the body to relax deeply while the mind remains inwardly alert. Yoga nidra is perfect in the evening to slow down that race car and bridge the gap between waking and sleep. It allows your brain to get into the same delta brainwave state as deep sleep. It is worth noting that traditionally yoga nidra was not used to help sleep but for deep relaxation and as a catalyst for achieving samadhi, a thoughtless state similar to nirvana or enlightenment in Buddhist philosophy. I like it because it is a path to hypnagogic sleep and lucid dreaming. More on that in Chapter 12.

But for now, we are going to aim for each session to last around twenty minutes. You don't want to read a script; you want to relax. Picture two buckets for this: five to ten minutes of preparation and ten to fifteen for visualization. If you want you can have someone help you through this or if you are worried about messing it up or forgetting something, practice when you go to bed at night, in the dark. This is also a helpful exercise when you can't sleep at night, so perfecting this is a valuable tool in your insomnia toolbox. There isn't a specific script for this, which is why I like it so much. Once you get the recipe down, make the recipe yours and yours alone.

Lie back in your bed and close your eyes – your back works the best but get comfortable. You need to not move for twenty minutes, so before you start, yes, pee, get a drink of water, anything that might distract you. Relax your body and mind as much as you can. You must stay as still as possible for the next twenty minutes or so. If you feel an itch or compulsion to move, try to refocus on your practice – each time you move will set you back a little.

Preparation is about connecting with your body, your mind, and your breath. It is easy to be so focused on our thoughts that we take our body for granted. Swirling thoughts, anxiety, and stress can be controlled and soothed by re-connecting with our bodies. Direct your awareness to your body, part by part.

Start with your neck and shoulders. How do they feel? Sense the tension in your muscles and allow it to dissipate. You may be surprised at how much tension you are holding; now is the time to be aware. Then move to your back and do the same thing. Next your face, your arms, and your legs. After taking an inventory of your body and tightening and released each one, it's time to move inward – to our emotions and thoughts. Take your time, there isn't time here. We want to separate from that clock that runs our day and picture our body tensing and relaxing, each part getting its turn. Allow yourself to recognize any major emotional or life events that are occurring at the moment.

Next, you will take inventory of your thoughts and emotions. This is brain dump 101. We are not trying to drain our thoughts away, like water out of a bathtub. We are recognizing and clearing them by looking at each piece and then putting it aside. I picture myself looking at all of the thoughts and emotion on my desk: they are a cluttered mess at the end of the day. I need to file them to clean off my desk. This is a physical process that your mind goes through during deep sleep. All of our "files" are kept in the hypothalamus until deep sleep and our brain files them then. You are just presorting, so it is easier during sleep. We want to get the emotional charge off of those files. We're often taught that meditation is about "emptying your mind." We aren't looking for empty, if thoughts are still in there and your brain isn't floating in oblivion, you are still good. Don't feel guilty for having thoughts. Mindfulness is more about how you react to your thoughts. Each thought has an emotional charge. Maybe on a scale of 1 to 10 it is low: for example, I need to get a haircut soon. But it can also have a big charge or lots of stress: for example, maybe a project you need to finish or a problem you need to solve. But as your thoughts pass by, another visual is in a river, you watch them go by, peaceful, and your emotional charge as an observer is significantly less.

Now it's time to bring ourselves fully into the present by refocusing awareness on our breath. Breathe naturally. Calmly.

Allow each breath to slowly fill you up. Maybe you have your hand on your belly, and you feel it rise. But don't move it there if it didn't start there or if you aren't comfortable with it resting there. Focus your awareness on these breaths, feel every detail of them. One by one. Where is it in your body? How does it feel? Is it a long breath or a short breath? Consider that every single breath is as different as the grains of sand on a beach. These grains of sand were once shells and rocks, and they have been tumbled by the ocean down to this size and place and time. Have each of your breaths become a simple part of you. This focus will actually change HRV, or heart rate variability. You are releasing stress out with every exhale. Start with breaths that can release that stress carried on the carbon dioxide back to the air, and then as the stress in your breath begins to decrease, recognize where in the body that breath is. Truly appreciate each breath. You are alive because of those breaths. Focus only on the breath. Allow any thoughts that intrude to flow away like water in the flowing stream. If thoughts are persistent, try counting the breaths or name them.

We are looking for a total of thirty breaths, but if it has been stressful and you need more, only you know how long you need for each body, mind, and breath section. Take your time. This is as good for you as sleep, so you aren't missing anything if this bites into your sleep window.

You should now be in a calm, relaxed, and "half-asleep" state. Your mind is alert, but your body is deeply relaxed and preparing for sleep. You are now ready to commence your yoga nidra visualizations.

You are lying on your back on a cloud, floating on top of a vast motionless ocean of blue sky. The cloud is soft and comfortable, and you feel safe, at peace and protected. The air is cool and refreshing, like a warm autumn day as you feel the steady stream of sunlight smiling down on your face and body. It looks like when the sun pokes through the clouds to shine down in streams of light. If the thought of God, the universe, or a benevolent force is shining on you, then bask in the warmth of that glow.

You are happy and comfortable, drifting on your back – with your eyes closed, safe, cased all around by your bubble of cloud and nothing is near your blanket of clouds. Rest here, drifting happily – without a care in the world. As you drift – content, warm, safe and protected – your awareness begins to fade away, and you drift off to sleep.

You may over time change the cloud to a place that feels safe for you. I like clouds because if thoughts, emotions, or pain tries to intrude, I blow them away on the fluffy clouds.

Sleep Aids

Many studies are finding that people who take prescription sleeping pills – even once in a while – have a higher death risk than those who do not. The top third of sleeping pill users had a 5.3-fold higher death risk and are linked to 320,000 to 507,000 US deaths each year. They also had a 35 percent higher risk of cancer, the study found.[62] "We are not certain. But it looks like sleeping pills could be as risky as smoking cigarettes. It looks much more dangerous to take these pills than to treat insomnia another way," said study leader Daniel F. Kripke, MD.

Prescription sleeping pills, like Ambien, are known as hypnotics. They include newer drugs such as zolpidem (Ambien) as well as older drugs such as temazepam (the best-known brand name is Restoril), eszopiclone (Lunesta), zaleplon (Sonata), triazolam (Halcion), and flurazepam (Dalmane). Hypnotic sleeping pills actually cause a person to fall asleep. This sets them apart from other sleeping aids, such as the supplement melatonin, which promote sleep through relaxation. The antihistamine such as diphenhydramine (Benedryl, NyQuil) is another over-the-counter one.

Sleep pills as hypnotics are best for people with acute, short episodes of insomnia.[63] The long-term safety of these drugs has never been studied. Over-the-counter sleep aids, like NyQuil or Aleve PM, can be effective for an occasionally sleepless night. They almost all contain antihistamines. Tolerance to the sedative effects of antihistamines can develop quickly – so the longer you take them, the less likely they are to make you sleepy. In addition, some over-the-counter sleep aids can leave you feeling groggy and unwell the next day, the sleep aid hangover. Doxylamine succinate (Unisom, Sleep Tabs) is also an antihistamine. Melatonin is the hormone that helps control your natural sleep/wake cycle. Some research suggests that melatonin supplements might be helpful in treating jet lag or reducing the time it takes to fall asleep – although the effect is typically mild. But again, no research on the long-

---

[62] Kripke, Daniel F. "What do hypnotics cost hospitals and healthcare?." *F1000Research* 6 (2017).

[63] Grewal, Ritu G., and Karl Doghramji. "Epidemiology of insomnia." *Clinical handbook of insomnia*. Springer, Cham, 2017. 13-25.

term effects, especially on children, has been conducted. When you replace a natural hormone for a long time, it usually causes problems that we just don't know yet. Valerian is an herbal supplement made from a plant that is sometimes taken as asleep aid. Although a few studies indicate some therapeutic benefit, other studies haven't found the same benefits. But at least valerian generally doesn't appear to cause side effects.

Cannabis is an interesting new player. It contains over 480 different compounds. CBD for healing is everywhere, and like most sleep aids, I am worried most people don't fully understand how it works – the how, when, or why. THC and CBD are pretty commonly talked about. THC is the part of cannabis that gets you high. You need a content of 5 percent or more to get high. CBD, which has been approved by the FDA for the treatment of epilepsy and only that, gets the credit for lots of therapeutic benefits. There is another one you should know, especially if you're considering CBD for sleep, called Terpenes.[64] Terpenes are what gives an orange its citrusy smell. They give pine trees their unique aroma and cause the relaxing effects of lavender. There are over 20,000 different terpenes in existence, and cannabis contains more than 100. Myrcene (also found in mangos) is the primary terpene found in cannabis plants, giving marijuana its distinctive aroma and relaxing and anti-inflammatory properties. Limonete (also found in citrus) may not be present in all cannabis strains. Limonene has powerful antifungal and antibacterial properties. Pinene (also found in pine trees) is a strong bronchodilator but also has strong anti-inflammatory and antiseptic effects. Linalool (also found in lavender) is

---

[64] Baron, Eric P. "Medicinal properties of cannabinoids, terpenes, and flavonoids in cannabis, and benefits in migraine, headache, and pain: an update on current evidence and cannabis science." *Headache: The Journal of Head and Face Pain* 58.7 (2018): 1139-1186.

widely known for its stress-relieving, anti-anxiety, and anti-depressant effect. Caryophyllene (found in cinnamon and black pepper) is capable of performing the big job of treating anxiety, depression, and inflammation. These are all examples of terpenes found in cannabis. When you get relief from using an oil, vaping, or putting on CBD lotions, it is a combination of all these. Just like every variety of apple has different taste, crunch, sweetness, color, and so on, cannabis strains do too. Finding out what is the right thing for you maybe a tricky process. It is also why some people will benefit and others won't. Just like two people won't react the same way to tasting an apple, it will be the same for a cannabis treatment. It boils down to trusting the chemist behind the product and then finding the right strain for what you need.

Confused yet? Yeah, me too. Terpenes can intensify or downplay the effects of the cannabinoids. Have you ever noticed how two similar strains can produce profoundly different effects? One may leave you with couch lock and the other may energize you. That's another aspect of the entourage effect, which is driven by both cannabinoids and terpenes. The heat from vaping can harm terpenes, so if you are hoping for a particular terpene effect, be careful how you consume your cannabis. There are hundreds of cannabis cultivars available to consumers, each with its own unique terpene and cannabinoid profile. Until you have tried a cultivar, you won't know how it will impact you. To cannabis use before bed or to help with sleep disorders, checking for mycene, linalool, and a-pinene, known for its anxiolytic effects, is a great place to start. Strains high in myrcene are often easiest to find because it is the most common terpene found in cannabis. This could include variants of Sour Diesel or OG Kush, like Platinum OG.

It may be the physicist in me that is weary of chemicals for sleep, but the efficacy of interventions, especially over time, is clear.

Use them to "cheat" for a night or to reset jet lag, but you can't just take a pill to sleep or you wouldn't be reading this book. Cannabis and all chemical interventions should be vetted for you, your body, and your situation.

How Much Sleep Do You Need?

This is probably one of the most common questions I get asked. You've probably read over and over again that a good night's rest equals eight hours of sleep. But research shows it's not the number of hours you sleep that matters the most – it's the quality of the hours you get. The largest sleep study ever conducted studied 1.1 million people and shows that it's quality, not quantity, that matters most. The researchers found that participants who slept only six and a half hours a night lived longer than those who slept eight hours. I think it is a question of quality, and that is why I am writing this book. It is in part because I feel that putting out one number for everyone is impossible; all 8 billion plus of us are not likely to be the same in how much sleep we need. In a hunter-gather research study on sleep, Jerome Siegel, leader of the research team and professor of psychiatry at UCLA's Semel Institute of Neuroscience and Human Behavior, found that they stay up late into the evening, average less than six and a half hours of sleep, and rarely nap[65]. The other fun fact he discovered was that people studied consistently slept during the nightly period of declining ambient temperature (back to the sleep switch and temperature). Insomnia was so rare among those studied that the San and the Tsimane do not have a word for insomnia at all.

---

[65] Yetish, Gandhi, Hillard Kaplan, and Michael Gurven. "Sleep variability and nighttime activity among Tsimane forager-horticulturalists." *American journal of physical anthropology* 166.3 (2018): 590-600.

Light

There are all kinds of light. I personally hate the light from LEDs and florescent lights, even during the day. Junk light – the blue light that emits from your smartphone, laptop, and tablet screens – is a mean culprit in destroying sleep. This infamous blue light can mess with your brain's production of melatonin. Blue light tells your brain that it's daytime.[66] Screens aren't the only source of junk light – streetlamps and those horrible but energy efficient LED lightbulbs are also to blame. Different people respond differently to blue light. I need a completely dark room; I have tried blue light glasses but am not sure they had much effect. But just like some people aren't affected by caffeine, some people might find that blue light is not a factor for them. Light is a valuable and potentially pivotal intervention. Plan to experiment with it during your first month.

What Should I Eat to Help Me Sleep?

Diet is tied to your sleep as well.[67] Your brain is the fattiest organ in the body and wants high-quality fats like grass-fed butter and wild-caught fish to nourish it so it can repair itself while you sleep. Filling up on fat at dinner means you're less likely to find yourself poking around the fridge at midnight. MCT oil before bedtime, blended into herbal tea, like a sleepy time tea, might help as well. But the best is to eat heavier earlier in the day, so have lunch be the biggest meal of the day.

---

[66] Shechter, Ari, et al. "Blocking nocturnal blue light for insomnia: A randomized controlled trial." *Journal of psychiatric research* 96 (2018): 196-202.

[67] Partinen, Markku. "Nutrition and sleep." *Sleep Disorders Medicine.* Springer, New York, NY, 2017. 539-558.

Vitamins, Minerals, and Other Hacks

Some of this could fall into the discussion on sleep aids, but some of these have efficacy because we are chronically short on them in our diets today. These are suggestions and supplements that enhance or exist in your body already.

Magnesium is one mineral we are chronically short on, by as much as 75 percent of the population.[68] It is hard to diagnose. It's a mineral that's crucial to the proper functioning of over 300 biochemical reactions in the body.[69] If you crave salty things, it can be a sign you need more magnesium and not having enough can stop you from getting to sleep. Another way to tell you are magnesium deficient is leg cramps, and it has been tied to restless leg syndrome. There are tablet supplements available; go for more than 400mg. But I like it best in a powder to put in a drink or, even better, as an oil for the bottoms of my feet. You can also take an Epsom salt bath before turning in for the night.

Potassium, the stuff in bananas, goes well with magnesium; the combination will remove nighttime leg cramps for most people. Fewer cramps equals more sleep[70]. There is such a thing as too much potassium, though. Take 400mg of potassium citrate at bedtime. Start with 100 to 200 and work your way up from there if you feel you need more.

---

[68] Weiss, Decker, Debra K. Brunk, and Dennis A. Goodman. "Scottsdale magnesium study: absorption, cellular uptake, and clinical effectiveness of a timed-release magnesium supplement in a standard adult clinical population." *Journal of the American College of Nutrition* 37.4 (2018): 316-327.

[69] McMillan, Joanna. "Health and wellbeing: The power of magnesium." LSJ: *Law Society of NSW Journal* 50 (2018): 54

[70] Yoshida, Kensuke, et al. "Leak potassium channels regulate sleep duration." *Proceedings of the National Academy of Sciences* 115.40 (2018): E9459-E9468.

L-theanine can come in capsule form or sometimes in teas and can help with relaxation. I would start with 100mg at night for a tablet.[71]

Chamomile tea actually does help you sleep. [72]But there is evidence that even hot water can have similar effects. Adding a tea at night is worthwhile. My favorite is Sleepy Time.it has chamomile in it.

GABA is a neuro-inhibitory transmitter. It helps your brain to shut itself down. It will dramatically calm you when you take it without any other proteins. Start with 500mg. GABA can also be taken midmorning during stressful times, but for most of us, nighttime use is best.

5-htp can easily enter your brain and create the happy hormone serotonin and release mood-lifting and sleep-inducing brain chemicals.[73] You will need to take breaks with this one or use as needed because you can build up a tolerance.

Activated charcoal can help reduce inflammation in your brain that maybe messing with your sleep. It can help by removing toxins from the gut before they reach your brain.

Vitamin D is deficient in more than half the world's population.[74] Low levels are linked with poor-quality sleep. You can get it naturally from the sun. But to get this important hormone (yes,

---

[71] Kim, Suhyeon, et al. "GABA and l-theanine mixture decreases sleep latency and improves NREM sleep." *Pharmaceutical biology* 57.1 (2019): 64-72.

[72] Jones, Kim. *222 Ways to Trick Yourself to Sleep: Scientifically Supported Ways to Fall Asleep and Stay Asleep.* Hachette UK, 2019.

[73] Hong, Ki-Bae, Yooheon Park, and Hyung Joo Suh. "Sleep-promoting effects of the GABA/5-HTP mixture in vertebrate models." *Behavioural brain research* 310 (2016): 36-41.

[74] van Schoor, Natasja, and Paul Lips. "Worldwide vitamin D status." *Vitamin D.* Academic Press, 2018. 15-40.

vitamin D is actually a hormone[75]), you should expose your skin to natural sunlight for about fifteen minutes per day, eat vitamin D-rich foods, and supplement with a high-quality vitamin D3.

Krill oil is full of brain-boosting omega-3 fatty acids.[76] Oily fish like sardines, krill, and salmon have it naturally. Some research shows it improves sleep and helps you fall asleep faster. The best way for this is to eat at least three servings of fatty fish a week. There are also tablets, although these can make your mouth taste fishy; if you use these, take 1,560mg of omega 3s twice a day, with meals.

I could go from here. There are more tips from traditional Chinese medicine, such as cup of chrysanthemum tea that clears heat (excessive yang energy) in the liver and calms the nerves. You can add goji berries to balance the chrysanthemum's inherent yin properties and to help nourish the liver. Jujube seed (suan zao ren) is commonly prescribed to treat insomnia.[77] It strengthens circulation and calms the mind, making you less irritable and restless. You can steep jujube seeds in hot water to drink it as a tea. The list seems endless it, which is why coming up with a plan and not trying to add too many things at once is important. Ayurveda is literally "the science of life" and actually predates TCM. Even the Greeks studied Ayurveda text. Ayurveda is synergetic with chronotype, so it is worth exploring how a deeper dive might benefit you.

---

[75] Gallo, Daniela, et al. "The story of a vitamin for bone health that upgraded to hormone for systemic good health." *Med Hist* 2 (2018): 152-160.

[76] Mosconi, Lisa. *Brain Food: How to Eat Smart and Sharpen Your Mind.* Penguin UK, 2018.

[77] Shergis, Johannah Linda, et al. "Ziziphus spinosa seeds for insomnia: a review of chemistry and psychopharmacology." *Phytomedicine* 34 (2017): 38-43.

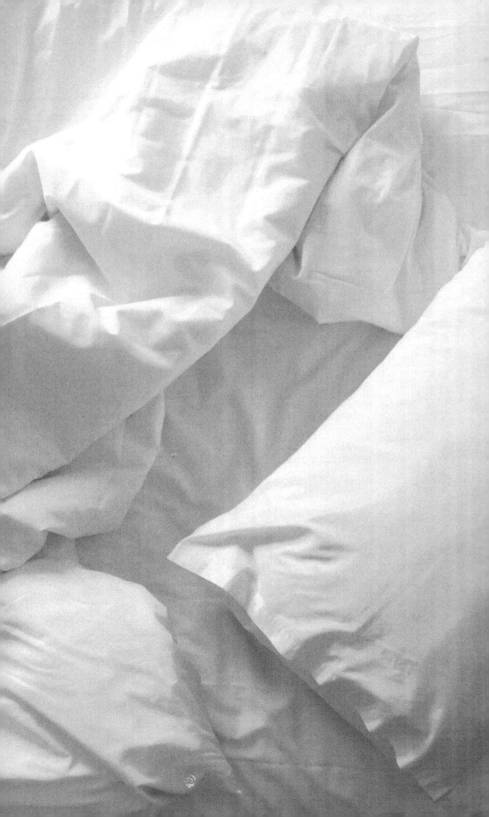

CHAPTER 10

Sleep Superpowers Activated

"The quality of a person's life is in direct proportion to their commitment to excellence, regardless of their chosen field of endeavor."

— Vince Lombardi —

There are many of reasons you have sleep problems. Some people are predisposed to get insomnia. This may mean that genetics is part of the equation, and you inherited it from your parents or family tree. It maybe from a life experience or experiences that disrupted your circadian rhythm and/or ideal hormone levels. It can be from both, like me. Your unique self with this weakness for insomnia is still capable of great things and this book is all about screaming from the rooftops to stop letting this weakness ruin and affect your life. Take back your sleep and you will be able to find what you are truly capable of. What does that mean? What are the goals I want to put out there as carrots? When you can recognize where sleep is holding you back and create a positive goal to work from, you can target this sleep thing most effectively. Reward yourself. Be clear what those will be. Tie it to specific metrics. How can you measure and quantify success if the goal and rewards are not clearly defined?

Memory

David graduated from Harvard and taught English for many years. He was a fabulous teacher, with great skill at sculpting lessons to truly reach his students. He has masses of literary memories in his head. In addition, there are all the other memories floating around. He pretty regularly shares them on Facebook for his fans to enjoy and heckle. But taking the liberty to speak on his behalf, he is worried about losing his cognitive wit and fortitude. I think we all are. If you consider yourself an intellectual at all, you treasure the web of references and contexts you have spent a lifetime to build.

But how does this hunk of gray matter represent and contain all of these memories and their needed references and context? You can remember your childhood home for example. There are likely a combination of unique memories and general ones. The individual ones do not exist separately from the more general ones. It is not known how activity patterns in the brain support the link between specific and general features of experience, which is necessary to correctly embed individual memories in broader knowledge structures. The hippocampus and prefrontal cortex (PFC) are thought to play complementary roles in maintaining these types of knowledge. We also generally know that while you sleep, your brain is busy processing information from the day and forming memories.[78] Events from the day are held in the hypothalamus and then sorted over a revolving approximate two-week window to decide what stays and what goes. For example, what you ate last Tuesday probably fell onto the cutting room floor, unless something meaningful happened, like you broke up with your boyfriend.

---

[78] Stickgold, Robert. "Sleep-dependent memory consolidation." *Nature* 437.7063 (2005): 1272-1278.

So how can we use this information to set goals for sleep? When you are tired, thought processes decrease, causing it to become nearly impossible to commit anything to memory. Lack of sleep will negatively impact learning anything new. Without an adequate amount of sleep, your brain has a difficult time absorbing and recalling new information. We do know sleep has an effect on the part of the brain where long-term memories are stored. Sleeping better should boost memories but what would I suggest for someone like Uncle David? Well, first we will consider his age – we will keep the exact number as a secret he can share for himself, but let's say past retirement. As you age, you lose deep sleep.[79] At twenty, we most likely had two hours of the eight be deep sleep, but by eighty you may be getting none. This is not good news for Uncle David.

A healthy human brain is made of tens of billions of neurons – specialized cells that process and transmit information using electrical and chemical signals. Neurons send messages between different parts of the brain, and from the brain to the muscles and organs of the body. In memory-related diseases like Alzheimer's, communication is disrupted among neurons and they lose functionality and die.[80] Unlike many cells in the body, which are relatively short-lived, neurons have evolved to live a long time – more than 100 years in humans. This means that, neurons must constantly be maintaining and repairing.

In a process called neurogenesis, adult brains may even generate new neurons. Remodeling of synaptic connections and neurogenesis

---

[79] Mander, Bryce A., Joseph R. Winer, and Matthew P. Walker. "Sleep and human aging." *Neuron* 94.1 (2017): 19-36.

[80] Schindowski, Katharina, et al. "Alzheimer's disease-like tau neuropathology leads to memory deficits and loss of functional synapses in a novel mutated tau transgenic mouse without any motor deficits." *The American journal of pathology* 169.2 (2006): 599-616.

are important for learning, memory, and possibly brain repair.[81] The aging brain may shrink to some degree in healthy aging but, surprisingly, does not loose neurons in large numbers. In a disease like Alzheimer's, many neurons stop functioning, loose connections with other neurons, and die. Alzheimer's disrupts processes vital to neurons and their networks, including communication, metabolism, and repair.

Recent studies suggest that Alzheimer's-related brain changes may result from an unusually high amount of abnormal tau proteins[82] among other factors. It appears that abnormal tau accumulates in specific brain regions involved in memory. Elevated tau is a sign of Alzheimer's disease and has been linked to brain damage and cognitive decline. "The key is that it wasn't the total amount of sleep that was linked to tau, it was the slow-wave sleep, which reflects quality of sleep,"[83] Brendan Lucey, MD, an assistant professor of neurology and director of the Washington University Sleep Medicine Center, stated. "The people with increased tau pathology were actually sleeping more at night and napping more in the day, but they weren't getting as good quality sleep." The best way I have heard to describe how deep sleep helps to prevent neurological diseases is our nightly deep sleep washes our brain[84]. Yep, a brain wash. At the start of healthy deep sleep, spinal fluid washes over your brain removing and managing toxin build ups. When the brain is deprived

---

[81] Mu, Yangling, and Fred H. Gage. "Adult hippocampal neurogenesis and its role in Alzheimer's disease." *Molecular neurodegeneration* 6.1 (2011): 85.

[82] Crimins, Johanna L., et al. "The intersection of amyloid beta and tau in glutamatergic synaptic dysfunction and collapse in Alzheimer's disease." *Ageing research reviews* 12.3 (2013): 757-763.

[83] Bhandari, Writer Tamara. "Decreased Deep Sleep Linked to Early Signs of Alzheimer's Disease." *Washington University School of Medicine in St. Louis*, 21 Jan. 2019, medicine. wustl.edu/news/decreased-deep-sleep-linked-to-early-signs-of-alzheimers-disease/.

[84] Boston University. "Are we 'brainwashed' during sleep? Cerebrospinal fluid washes in and out of brain during sleep." *ScienceDaily.* ScienceDaily, 31 October 2019.

of deep sleep for long periods of time, tau builds up. The deep sleep brain wash is one of the ways that deep sleep can help David and one of the key superpowers we can hope to gain from getting better sleep.

I have found that deep sleep over time does have recovery benefits for brain fog and short-term memory. This is superpower worthy. Researchers from the Washington University study hope to be able to use a sleep quality metric as a predictor for Alzheimer's. Putting on your deep sleep armor may not make you bullet proof to memory loss, but it gets pretty close. Bam. First new superpower.

Organize, Focus, Decision-Making

Sleep helps your brain function. Remember Susan from Chapter 1? She is a great example of what six months of great sleep can do. Morning is supposed to be the most productive part of your day. But when you are sleep deprived, you exist in this limbo between should I stay under the covers and just keep trying and if I hurry up, I can get my day over with and try again tonight. A sleep study by the Rand Institute found that "sleep deprivation is linked to lower productivity at work, which results in a significant amount of working days being lost each year. On an annual basis, the U.S. loses an equivalent of around 1.2 million working days due to insufficient sleep. This is followed by Japan, which loses on average 600,000 working days per year. The UK and Germany both lose just over 200,000 working days. Canada loses around 80,000 working days.[85]" The global sleep epidemic is costing the world's economies billions of dollars every year. The US economy has the largest loss, with an estimated $411 billion annually through tired or absent employees.

---

[85] "The Costs of Insufficient Sleep." *RAND Corporation*, www.rand.org/randeurope/research/projects/the-value-of-the-sleep-economy.html.

The Enormous Cost Of Sleep Deprivation
Estimated annual cost of insufficient sleep in GDP terms (billion U.S. dollars)*

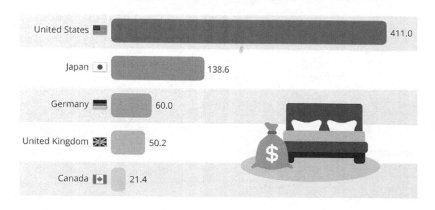

United States	411.0
Japan	138.6
Germany	60.0
United Kingdom	50.2
Canada	21.4

* Highest estimate - due to loss of productivity
@StatistaCharts Source: RAND

statista

How a person can engage in activity is limited by a physiological maximal processing capacity. Just like the processing capacity of a computer, if you have low capacity, you aren't going to process information effectively. Information processing of differing types requires varying levels of attention and engagement and each makes unique demands us from moment to moment. Effort can be looked at as an attempt by the brain to meet the needs presented. When the processor isn't working as we need it to, there is increased time on tasks.

Staying on top of your game and going the extra mile are great, but if you are tired, it just doesn't work. Getting more done is a superpower. As a parent, you are always juggling, and there isn't enough time so getting more done. Sounds super to me. Think of a project that needs organizing or problem solving. With sleep, you can accomplish it, so put it out there. When I am tired, I become lazy. I struggle to stay on top of household tasks like laundry and even sorting and filing my email lags behind. What will be your productivity goal?

Energized

Having a house full of boys means that Stars Wars is a part of my life. One year, the boys all dressed up as Star Wars characters. In the 1999 film Episode 1: The Phantom Menace, George Lucas introduces us to "midi-chlorians." They give some characters the ability to sense and use the Force. They are the source of our inner power. George Lucas himself described them as "a loose depiction of mitochondria." Mitochondria are the power source inside all your body's cells. They are organelles, (basically like an organ inside a cell) that act like your digestive system for your cells, taking in nutrients, breaking them down, and creating energy-rich molecules for the cell called adenosine triphosphate, or ATP. The biochemical processes of the cell are known as cellular respiration.

Fun fact: Mitochondria have their own set of DNA[86] and mitochondrial DNA (mtDNA) is more similar to bacterial DNA and comes from your mother. As you probably know, half of a child's DNA comes from his or her father and half from his or her mother. The child always receives their mtDNA from their mother. For instance, mtDNA analyses have concluded that humans may have originated in Africa relatively recently, around 200,000 years ago, descended from a common ancestor, known as mitochondrial Eve.

As you grow older, your body has fewer mitochondria. "If you feel you don't have enough energy, it can be because your body has problems producing enough ATP and thus providing cells with enough energy[87]," says Dr. Anthony Komaroff, professor of medicine at Harvard Medical School. During deep sleep, ATP levels

---

[86] Fleming, J. E., et al. "Is cell aging caused by respiration-dependent injury to the mitochondrial genome?." *Gerontology* 28.1 (1982): 44-53.

[87] Harvard Health Publishing. "Refueling Your Energy Levels." *Harvard Health*, 2018, www.health.harvard.edu/staying-healthy/refueling-your-energy-levels.

surge.[88] It is one of the key functions of sleep to maintain energy balance in the brain. The health of our mitochondria determines the amount of ATP they can produce from the calories we eat and oxygen we consume. Without robust mitochondria, cells cannot do as much work as they're capable of and we need them to do so we can stay healthy. One of the main mechanisms that makes sleep so important for mitochondrial health is the "glymphatic system,[89]" which was described in a 2018 report. Restorative sleep allows the brain to clear the byproducts of thinking (waste) and maintain healthful mitochondria[90].

So being energized is certainly a sleep superpower. With more energy, will you play more, heal more, do more? What goals will you set for your more energized self?

Be Motivated

After Benjamin died, I became a mild hoarder. I couldn't get rid of anything. Not only was it emotionally stressful, but I failed to be motivated to do anything about it. Fortunately, it took the form of an extremely cluttered attic. Emotionally, I couldn't part with any toy or outgrown piece of clothing. It was a vicious cycle where my relatively organized self, when I am rested and healthy, felt guilt and shame for not cleaning up. And on the other side, my exhausted, grief-ridden self, just didn't have the emotional energy to tackle it.

---

[88] Aalling, Nadia Nielsen, Maiken Nedergaard, and Mauro DiNuzzo. "Cerebral metabolic changes during sleep." *Current neurology and neuroscience reports* 18.9 (2018): 57.

[89] Plog, Benjamin A., and Maiken Nedergaard. "The glymphatic system in central nervous system health and disease: past, present, and future." *Annual Review of Pathology: Mechanisms of Disease* 13 (2018): 379-394.

[90] Nicolson, Garth L., et al. "Mitochondrial Dysfunction and Chronic Disease: Treatment with Membrane Lipid Replacement and Other Natural Supplements." *Mitochondrial Biology and Experimental Therapeutics*. Springer, Cham, 2018. 499-522.

Perhaps that is an extreme case, but it is not unusual for depression and mental health to degrade with sleep deprivation. It could be as simple as not feeling like doing the dishes in the sink. It could be putting off a diet, exercise program, and trip.

I don't think it is surprising that lack of sleep is connected to our self-control. Those late-night tired hungries are due to not having the willpower to resist the temptation. Having good self-control requires a lot of effort, which wilts away when you are sleep deprived. Thus, without the energy for willpower, people who are sleep deprived tend to gain weight. A group led by Drs. Erin Hanlon and Eve Van Cauter at the University of Chicago wanted to better understand how sleep and weight gain interact biologically. They noticed that sleep deprivation has effects in the body similar to activation of the endocannabinoid (eCB) system, a key player in the brain's regulation of appetite and energy levels. Perhaps most well-known for being activated by chemicals found in marijuana, famously known as "the munchies."[91] The eCB system affects the brain's motivation and reward circuits and can spark a desire for fast and high-carb foods.

According to Sanjay Patel, a professor at the Critical Care and Sleep Medicine at Western University, poor sleep is linked to both present and future obesity.[92] Without being well rested, it is difficult to control temptations for junk food and have the willpower to exercise. In order to function properly, your brain requires a good amount of glucose. However, when you're tired, your brain quickly exhausts your glucose reserves and is not able to absorb or replenish them properly. When your brain realizes it's lacking glucose, the

[91] Hanlon, Erin C., et al. "Sleep restriction enhances the daily rhythm of circulating levels of endocannabinoid 2-arachidonoylglycerol." *Sleep* 39.3 (2016): 653-664.

[92] Ogilvie, Rachel P., and Sanjay R. Patel. "The epidemiology of sleep and obesity." *Sleep Health* 3.5 (2017): 383-388.

craving for simple carbs, sugar, and caffeine begins. The researchers found that the sleep deprived consumed on average an extra 385 calories per day–which can lead to weight gain.[93] Two hormones that help regulate hunger–ghrelin and leptin–are affected by sleep: Ghrelin stimulates your hunger urge while leptin decreases it. When the body is sleep deprived, the level of ghrelin spikes, while the level of leptin falls, leading to an increase in hunger.[94]

So maybe your superpower goal is to lose weight? Remember a goal like losing weight comes after you get your superpowers and are ready to tackle things like diet. For me it was finally getting my house in order, in both a literal and figurative way.

Control Emotions

When I think about controlling emotions, I picture the Snickers advertisement where Betty White is playing football. She is snippy and slow. The Snickers bar turns her back into herself. You are Betty White when you are sleep deprived. You, however, are learning to sleep again and those superpowers are better than a chocolate bar. Sleep deprivation can lead to a state called "mild prefrontal dysfunction,[95]" during which your brain no longer has the ability to regulate your emotions or attention. During this state, you are Betty White. In all seriousness, sleep deprivation is attached to depression, anxiety, suicide rates, attention deficit hyperactivity disorder (ADHD), and every single mental illness. It's not a small thing.

---

[93] "A Good Night's Sleep Can Help You Maintain A Healthy Weight." *National Sleep Foundation,* www.sleepfoundation.org/excessive-sleepiness/health-impact/good-nights-sleep-can-help-you-maintain-healthy-weight.

[94] Young, John K. *Hunger, Thirst, Sex, and Sleep: How the Brain Controls Our Passions.* Rowman & Littlefield, 2016.

[95] Satterfield, B. C., et al. "0233 GABA: A Neural Marker of Resilience to Psychomotor Vigilance Impairment during Sleep Deprivation." *Sleep* 41 (2018): A90.

At Christmas time, National Lampoon's Christmas Vacation is always a hit. In one scene, Clark finds out his bonus was a subscription to the jelly of the month club, so the pool he was planning, and the check he wrote to reserve it, are now in trouble. He didn't get what he was promised. He launches into a physical tirade. Will is a lot like Clark. He calls it hopping mad. Although that anger hasn't hurt anybody, it can put a hole in a wall. Todd has struggled with managing business stress at different times. Anger and stress can simmer under the surface. You don't get angry because you are tired, but if you are angry or stressed, being tired allows it to come out and often in an uncontrolled way We discussed earlier, sleep makes decisions and managing thoughts difficult. Stress like financial or work pressure combined with sleep deprivation is toxic. You may find you need to handle the anger side parallel to the sleep recipe. Will had a mix of trauma, financial, work stress, and sleep deprivation. Todd had to handle his stress and manage his anger through a therapist but handling that amplified his success with his sleep.

Even small levels of sleep deprivation over time can chip away at your happiness, success, or loneliness – the list is endless. It can range from just being less enthusiastic or more irritable to even symptoms of clinical depression, such as feeling persistently sad or empty. It isn't just your individual mental health but your relationships dynamics as well. As stated by Harvard Health, "People with insomnia have greater levels of depression and anxiety than those who sleep normally. They are ten times as likely to have clinical depression and seventeen times as likely to have clinical anxiety. The more a person experiences insomnia and the more frequently they wake at night as a result, the higher the chances of developing depression."[96]

---

[96] Harvard Health Publishing. "Sleep and Mental Health." *Harvard Health*, 2019, www. health.harvard.edu/newsletter_article/sleep-and-mental-health.

A normal sleeper cycles between the major categories of sleep – although the length of time spent in one varies. Veterans and others with posttraumatic stress disorder (PTSD) often report suboptimal sleep quality, often described as lack of restfulness. Multiple studies suggest that patients with PTSD are deficient in deep and/or REM sleep[97], but particularly with a loss of deep sleep. Getting deep sleep is a big deal all around. We have ongoing studies with veterans. We donate more than $100,000 of product each year, in addition to funding studies on veterans and sleep. Early results showed that regulating temperature and matching it to the circadian rhythm is helping reduce episodes of PTSD. Hopefully a simple thing like temperature will be a big part of the equation for them.

Let's look ahead and say you are getting your required deep sleep. What are you going to do with all of that emotion strength? Maybe it is just being a better football player and less like Betty White. But it's okay to think big.

---

[97] Onton, Julie A., et al. "In-home sleep recordings in military veterans with post-traumatic stress disorder reveal less rem and deep sleep< 1 Hz." *Frontiers in human neuroscience* 12 (2018): 196.

CHAPTER 11

EMF? 5G? The Ghost in the Machine

"The greatest polluting element in the earth's environment is the proliferation of electromagnetic fields. I consider that to be a far greater threat on a global scale than warming, or the increase of chemical elements in the environment."
— Robert O. Becker —

In Gilbert Ryle's book *The Ghost in the Machine*, he tackles Descartes's mind-body split. This is not the book to debate that philosophy, but I like the visual image of a ghost in the machine. Electricity in our bodies is somewhat invisible and seems like a ghost. As everyday people, we are aware that lots of things happen inside our body. For the most part, this is governed by our lower school education. Digestion, muscles, breathing, and cardiovascular actions are pretty much understood in a basic sense. We don't have a good sense on how electrons flow in our bodies and biophysics in general. Most of this chapter focuses on the facts behind putting tin foil on your head, or chemical and electromagnetic sensitivity. I debated this chapter the most because it is an overall health issue we need to tackle as well, but one of the big symptoms of electromagnetic field (EMF) exposure is insomnia and depression. We are going to then take a brief interlude to look at what we can see that might be affecting your sleep. For some of you this will look like chasing ghosts. But you can't see gravity either, but it certainly affects us every day.

You may or may not have heard of EMFs. Remember to read this despite that fact you are getting flashbacks from the X-Files. You may be someone who believes in EMFs and maybe you think they are related to UFOs. I will make the case to believe and keep an open mind. I actually think that Wi-Fi and cell phones make these waves seem more real because like gravity we can see the results.

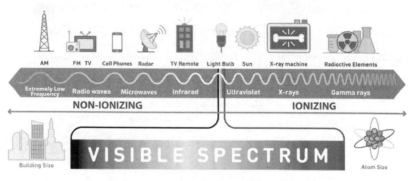

The electromagnetic spectrum. The narrow range of visible light is shown enlarged in the middle.

Encyclopædia Britannica, Inc.

An electromagnetic field (EMF) is a magnetic field produced by electrically charged objects. These energy fields surround us all the time. Scientists like to group things too, so they are organized by wavelength and frequency. There are two general kinds of electromagnetic radiation: ionizing radiation and nonionizing radiation.[98] Ionizing radiation is powerful enough to knock electrons

[98] The Editors of Encyclopaedia Britannica. "Electromagnetic Spectrum." *Encyclopædia Britannica*, Encyclopædia Britannica, Inc., 11 Mar. 2019, www.britannica.com/science/electromagnetic-spectrum.

out of their orbit around an atom. In the picture above you see radioactive elements are an example of this. This process is called ionization and can be damaging to a body's cells. Nonionizing radiation has enough energy to move atoms in a molecule around and cause them to vibrate, which makes the atom heat up, but not enough to remove the electrons from the atoms. As you can see light is a kind of EMF. There are four categories of EMFs that are linked to health outcomes: radio frequency (RF), magnetic fields (MF), electric fields (EF), and something called dirty electricity (DE)[99].

When electricity flows through a wire, or other metallic object, you get an electromagnetic field. It combines both MF and EF. MF from electricity in your house falls into 50Hz to 60Hz range (60Hz in North America and 50Hz in Europe). Still with me? Hang in there. Cell phones, Bluetooth, Wi-Fi are all RF. DE is all over the place ranging from 300Hz to 10MHz. Although EMF occur in nature, the bucket of EMF we now live with is messy and at levels much higher than that found in nature. Every smart device adds to this bucket. "We currently live in an environment estimated to contain more than 10 billion times more RF radiation than it did in the 1960s. If this environment is safe we're talking about in the order of 15,000 to 25,000 papers – in peer-reviewed scientific journals – all being wrong. That has never happened before,"[100] says an associate, a neuroscientist at the Karolinska Institute in Sweden

What does all of these mean to me? Magnetic fields affect the behavior of any other charged objects in the vicinity of the field.

[99] "Electromagnetic Fields and Public Health." *World Health Organization,* World Health Organization, 4 Aug. 2016, www.who.int/peh-emf/publications/facts/fs304/en/.

[100] Waters, Florence. "Is Wi-Fi Making Your Child Ill?" *The Telegraph,* Telegraph Media Group, 1 June 2017, www.telegraph.co.uk/health-fitness/body/wifi-internet-family-dangerous-health/.

Our bodies are electric. Your heartbeat generates electromagnetic waves throughout the blood vessels of the body, stimulating tissues at a cellular level. External magnetic fields and the normal electric and electromagnetic fields produced by the body interact. An EMF passing through your whole body will have an electromagnetic effect on each of your 70 trillion cells.[101]

A review of more than two dozen studies on low-frequency EMFs suggests that they may cause various neurological and psychiatric problems in people. This study found a link between EMF exposure and changes in human nerve function throughout the body, affecting things like sleep and mood.[102] When they look at cell phones there are guidelines for distances away from the body or specific absorption rate (SAR). It averages from 5mm for and Apple iPhone and up to 15mm for a Samsung. And yes, that is in the fine print. Now that isn't too far away, so it's not too bad, right? In your pocket isn't that far away. I fall into this trap as well. It is terribly convenient to have those darn things with us all the time. As I mentioned above, the effects of devices vary in frequency ranges, from extremely low frequencies (ELFs), to low frequencies (VLFs). When frequencies and intensities are high, like in the case of cell phones, power lines, and so on, it can induce heat in the tissues of the body and modify genes and, therefore, can damage cells.[103]

---

[101] Karimi, Seyed Asaad, et al. "Effects of exposure to extremely low-frequency electromagnetic fields on spatial and passive avoidance learning and memory, anxiety-like behavior and oxidative stress in male rats." *Behavioural brain research* 359 (2019): 630-638.

[102] Pritchard, Colin, Anne Silk, and Lars Hansen. "Are rises in Electro-Magnetic Field in the human environment, interacting with multiple environmental pollutions, the tripping point for increases in neurological deaths in the Western World?." *Medical hypotheses* 127 (2019): 76-83.

[103] Home, E. M. F. "History, research and health Implications of artificial EMFs." *History* (2019).

The cocoon of sleep is special for healing[104]. We have already covered that. During deep sleep, our body wants to detox and heal. We want less stress and less cortisol, but EMFs increase these. If sleep problems persist, it may be worth going down this rabbit hole. More and more studies link EMFs to health issues.[105] Just like caffeine and light, you will have to determine if this has an effect on you. But a study found that in general people slept 90 percent better without low EMFs.[106]

Michael has always struggled with depression. He also struggled with sleep. He has gone on meditations and yoga trips around the world. He has mastered advanced yoga and meditation techniques, and they have and do help with his depression and sleep. But he also lives in an apartment building in a city. In a TEDx talk on Wireless Wake-Up by Jeromy Johnson, he explores some of the effects that these Wi-Fi and wireless networks have on our bodies. Michael is sensitive to these.

Electromagnetic hypersensitivity (EHS) is a claimed sensitivity to electromagnetic fields, to which negative symptoms are attributed.[107] Science is not sure if wants to commit to a position on this. I feel like it is like the debate around climate change. There are natural ways in which climate is influenced, like volcanos and other natural phenomena, so we discount our role as also being a huge

---

[104] Hekmatmanesh, Amin, et al. "Bedroom design orientation and sleep electroencephalography signals." *Acta Medica International* 6.1 (2019): 33.

[105] Bagheri Hosseinabadi, Majid, et al. "The effect of chronic exposure to extremely low-frequency electromagnetic fields on sleep quality, stress, depression and anxiety." *Electromagnetic biology and medicine* 38.1 (2019): 96-101.

[106] Nasim, Imtiaz. "Analysis of Human EMF Exposure in 5G Cellular Systems." (2019).

[107] Dömötör, Zsuzsanna, et al. "Modern health worries: A systematic review." *Journal of psychosomatic research* 124 (2019): 109781.

factor. A river will naturally change course over time. We see lots of evidence for this. But building a dam makes a bigger change and a more significant one.

EMFs are absolutely having and will have an effect in the future. As humans we didn't have EMFs like we are producing today even twenty years ago. The effect for most people is lost in all the other ways and things going on, so we think that it's okay to discount and ignore them. For people like Michael, EMFs disturb his mind, his sleep, and his health. Like the other tips in this book, you will have decided what effect, if any, some of these factors have on you and your sleep. We are all different in what we are sensitive to.

Can an EMF Be Good?

Another example is the Earth's magnetic field. It is what we call a pulsing magnetic field. The Earth has its own magnetic fields, which are generated by fluxes in the molten metal in the outer core of the planet. These magnetic fields extend from the interior of the planet to where it meets the solar wind, which emanates from the Sun. It protects us from solar winds, which would otherwise destroy the protective ozone layer in our atmosphere. This magnetic field makes compasses work and is also used by pigeons and fish to navigate. Schumann resonance (SR) is the more specific way to describe the background stationary electromagnetic noise that propagates in the frequency range between 5Hz and 50Hz. The phenomenon was named after W. O. Schumann who first predicted and discussed it in 1950s. What I think is interesting for us, is that the first four SR modes happen to be match frequencies of brain waves during sleep (i.e., Delta [Deep Sleep] is 0.5–3.5Hz).[108]

---

[108] Zhang, Shujun, et al. "The Effects of Bio-inspired Electromagnetic Fields on Healthy Enhancement with Case Studies." *Emerging Science Journal* 3.6 (2019): 369-381.

PEMF, Pulsing Magnetic Fields? Where Did This Come From?

In 1898, Tesla published a paper that he read at the eighth annual meeting of the American Electro-Therapeutic Association in Buffalo, New York. He is one of my science heroes. In that paper, he becomes the first person to talk about PEMFs. In the 1960s, Robert O. Becker, in his book The Body Electric, establishes that the Chinese meridians of the body are skin pathways of decreased electrical resistance. Dr. Andrew Bassett, along with Dr. Arthur Pilla, developed an effective PEMF generator to stimulate bone fracture healing,[109] now approved by the FDA with an 80 percent success rate. Dr. Goodwin, manager of the Disease Modeling and Tissue Analogues Laboratory at the NASA Johnson Space Center and Lead Scientist for the Oxidative Stress and Damage, is known for his research into effects of PEMF and ultra-low frequency electromagnetic fields on human tissues.[110] It is actually a real thing.

Using PEMF for Sleep

A study, by Pawluk, found significant relief for insomnia with PEMF.[111] I have experimented with these as well, and they can work, although I would not say they should be the first line of interaction; I think more research needs to explore this. Maybe we can find a way to counteract EMF with PEMF.

---

[109] Prakash, Divya, Shikha S. Chauhan, and Jitendra Behari. "Therapeutic effectiveness of Hydroxyapatite Nanoparticles and Pulsed Electromagnetic Field in Osteoporosis and Cancer." (2019).

[110] Cottrill, Ethan, et al. "The effect of electrical stimulation therapies on spinal fusion: a cross-disciplinary systematic review and meta-analysis of the preclinical and clinical data." *Journal of Neurosurgery: Spine* 1.aop (2019): 1-21.

[111] Pawluk, W. "Pulsed Magnetic Field Treatment of Anxiety, Panic and Post-Traumatic Stress Disorders." *J Altern Complement Integr Med* 5 (2019): 075

Grounding

This is the practice of connecting with the earth. This is bare skin or bare feet on dirt, not concrete. Using the same science basics as above, our body's heart and brain, immune system, and other systems operate electrically. Grounding, or earthing, is about connecting our bodies to the Earth. Research shows that earthing generates major health benefits such as:

- Rapid reduction or elimination of chronic pain
- Dynamic blood flow improvement to better supply the cells and tissues of the body with vital oxygen and nutrition
- Reduced stress
- Increased energy
- Improved sleep
- Accelerated healing from injuries and surgery[112]

There are sheets and mats to help with grounding, and I feel there is absolutely an effect here. I wouldn't run out and get grounding but instead start with walking barefoot outside as part of your daily outside breaks. See if it makes a difference to you.

Acupuncture

Before you dismiss the idea of putting needles in your body, assume that all of this electricity stuff is real (I hope you do). Acupuncture has been shown to be effective in treating insomnia.[113] Acupuncture dates back to at least 100 BC, which is when an organized system of diagnosis and treatment using needles was first described

---

[112] Chevalier, Gaétan, et al. "The effects of grounding (earthing) on bodyworkers' pain and overall quality of life: A randomized controlled trial." *EXPLORE* 15.3 (2019): 181-190.

[113] He, Wenbo, et al. "Acupuncture for treatment of insomnia: An overview of systematic reviews." *Complementary therapies in medicine* 42 (2019): 407-416.

in writing in China. In traditional Chinese medicine, acupuncture is linked to the belief that disease is caused by disruptions to the flow of energy, or qi, in the body. Acupuncture uses needles placed strategically to help balance your flow of qi (or chi) throughout your body. Needles are placed in specific points along fourteen meridians – or qi pathways – in your body in order to rebalance your energy flow. When qi gets stuck, it can cause pain, discomfort, reduced bodily function, or illness. Acupuncture stimulates points on or under the skin called acupuncture points or acupressure points, releasing this qi. Acupuncture works through neurohormonal pathways. Basically, you put the needle through specific points in the body and stimulate the nerve. This applies specifically to dry needling. It is a technique employed by physical therapists and is similar in that a needle is inserted into the skin to alleviate pain. However, the primary difference between acupuncture and dry needling is that acupuncture treats for the purpose of altering the flow of qi (or energy) along traditional Chinese meridians while dry needling follows evidence-based guidelines, recommended "point" locations, and dosages for the treatment of specific conditions.

Research shows that dry needling improves pain control, reduces muscle tension[114], and normalizes dysfunctions of the motor end plates, the sites at which nerve impulses are transmitted to muscles. This can help speed up the patient's return to active rehabilitation.

I think acupuncture is more effective for sleep because it isn't just sticking a needle where there needs to be stimulation but is activating your parasympathetic system, the part of your nervous

---

[114] Pourahmadi, Mohammadreza, et al. "Effectiveness of dry needling for improving pain and disability in adults with tension-type, cervicogenic, or migraine headaches: protocol for a systematic review." *Chiropractic & manual therapies* 27.1 (2019): 43.

system that encourages your body to rest and digest. Acupuncture practitioners will use a conversational method to determine which points are most appropriate for you. An example may be between the shoulder blades around the heart level (B38: Vital Diaphragm) to reduce sleep stress. There are also specific meridians (qi pathways) tied to sleep, such as the heart meridian for sleep onset or the liver meridian if you are waking up hot in the middle of the night.[115] You may be sitting there questioning this whole thing. I get it, the science geek agrees. I use it for treatment in my lower back, in addition to cryotherapy – stay tuned. It helped one of my sons with bed wetting when the doctor basically said just leave it be and hope he grows out of it. The fourteen-year-old preferred needles; for this they go in the top of your head, so he could get past it. It, hands down, helped. It can do wonders in my opinion for sinus infections and of course sleep. But it, like everything else in this chapter, is okay to put into the maybe category.

Acupressure

Yes, this you can do at home.

Spirit Gate

Stimulating this pressure point is associated with quieting your mind, which can help you fall asleep[116].

1. Feel for the small, hollow space in this area and apply gentle pressure in a circular or up-and-down movement.

2. Continue for two to three minutes.

---

[115] Brobyn, Tracy L., Tia Trivisonno, and Patrick J. LaRiccia. "Challenging Case in Clinical Practice: Five Element Chinese Medicine Approach to Sleep Maintenance Insomnia." *Alternative and Complementary Therapies* 24.1 (2018): 10-12.

[116] Aygin, Dilek, and Sevim Şen. "Acupressure on Anxiety and Sleep Quality After Cardiac Surgery: A Randomized Controlled Trial." *Journal of PeriAnesthesia Nursing* 34.6 (2019): 1222-1231.

3. Hold the left side of the point with gentle pressure for a few seconds, and then hold the right side.

4. Repeat on the same area of your other wrist.

Frontier Gate

1. Turn your hands over so that your palms are facing up.

2. Take one hand and count three finger widths down from your wrist crease.

3. Apply a steady downward pressure between the two tendons in this location.

4. Use a circular or up-and-down motion to massage the area for four to five seconds.

Cryotherapy, Ice Baths, Saunas

Ice

Like I said before, I use a three-minute time out in a cryogenic chamber regularly for back pain. But cold and heat therapy can help with sleep as well.[117] Tim Ferriss has used ice baths before bed. According to "the Iceman," Wim Hof, "Over time, we, as humans have developed a different attitude towards nature around us and we actually forgot one thing, 'inner power.' This is the relationship by our physiological mechanisms to adapt and survive within our natural environment, which is direct and effective. Because we wear clothes and control the temperatures at home and work, we have changed the stimulation on our body, thus the old mechanisms related to survive and function. As these deeper physiological layers are not stimulated anymore, we have become alienated from them, thus our bodies have weakened, and we are no longer in touch with this inner power. The

---

[117] G. Banfi, G. Lombardi, A. Colombini, G. Melegati **Whole-body cryotherapy in athletes** Sports Med, 40 (2010), pp. 509-517

inner power is a force accumulated by full awakened physiological processes. It also influences the core of our DNA."[118]

"Wim Hof got his nickname "The Iceman" by breaking a number of records related to cold exposure. His feats include climbing Mount Kilimanjaro in shorts, running a half marathon above the Arctic Circle on his bare feet, and standing in a container while covered with ice cubes for more than 112 minutes", from his website, the wimhofmethod.com.

You can find many studies on the benefits of cold-water therapy, including weight loss stimulation, increased circulation, and stress reduction.[119] Taking a cold shower may even serve as a potential antidepressant, according to a 2008 study published by the National Institutes of Health. Does it help me sleep?[120] I can't unequivocally tie it to that, but it helps with stress, pain, and mental clarity for sure.

Saunas, Warm Baths, and Socks

If you have never visited a sauna before, you may not have considered the benefits saunas provide for your sleep routine. Going to the sauna can help you sleep better. This may not work if you don't have one in your house, but in countries like Finland, it is common. When I visited earlier this year, I tried it out, and I liked it. I do think I prefer cold therapy, but I have done that much longer. In addition, I found going to bed too hot was a problem so manage that as it makes sense to you. Saunas have been as part of a treatment for chronic fatigue syndrome[121].

---

[118] "Online Video Course." *Wim Hof Method*, explore.wimhofmethod.com/.

[119] Douzi, Wafa, et al. "3-min whole body cryotherapy/cryostimulation after training in the evening improves sleep quality in physically active men." *European journal of sport science* 19.6 (2019): 860-867.

[120] N.A. Shevchuk **Adapted cold shower as a potential treatment for depression** Med Hypotheses, 70 (2008), pp. 995-1001

[121] Bunnell, David E., et al. "Passive body heating and sleep: influence of proximity to sleep." *Sleep* 11.2 (1988): 210-219.

You see it in the online tips. Yes, putting on socks before bed can help. "A cool core and comfortably warm skin is best for sleep," said Roy Raymann, PhD, vice-president of sleep science at SleepScore Labs. Raymann has published research on the phenomenon in Physiology & Behavior about the efficacy of socks[122]. Feet have many temperature sensors; by warming them with socks, it may signal the brain to go to sleep. In a small study published in the Journal of Physiological Anthropology, subjects with socks took about half as long as those without socks to fall asleep.

Weighted Blankets

These are basically just like they sound. Blankets that are filled with plastic beads or pellets to make them heavier. They typically weigh from three pounds to twenty pounds. Typically, it is recommended that you buy one that weighs approximately 10 percent of your body weight, which would mean a 15-pound blanket for a 150-pound person. They can be a solution for insomnia as well as nighttime anxiety and stress reduction. And I agree. I love mine. The idea of using weight as a calming strategy does have some basis in current medical practice. "Weighted blankets have been around for a long time, especially for kids with autism or behavioral disturbances,[123]" says Dr. Cristina Cusin, an assistant professor of psychiatry at Harvard Medical School. "It is one of the sensory tools commonly used in psychiatric units. Patients who are in distress

---

[122] Raymann, Roy JEM, Dick F. Swaab, and Eus JW Van Someren. "Cutaneous warming promotes sleep onset." *American Journal of Physiology-Regulatory, Integrative and Comparative Physiology* 288.6 (2005): R1589-R1597.

[123] Harvard Health Publishing. "Anxiety and Stress Weighing Heavily at Night? A New Blanket Might Help." *Harvard Health*, 2019, www.health.harvard.edu/mind-and-mood/anxiety-and-stress-weighing-heavily-at-night-a-new-blanket-might-help.

may choose different types of sensory activities – holding a cold object, smelling particular aromas, manipulating dough, building objects, doing arts and crafts – to try to calm down. Weighted blankets feel like comforting hug, in theory helping to calm and settle the nervous system.

CHAPTER 12

Sleep Is a Journey

"And if tonight my soul may find her peace in sleep, and sink in good oblivion, and in the morning wake like a new-opened flower then I have been dipped again in God, and new-created."

– D. H. Lawrence –

We buy gym memberships and try it for a while and lose motivation. We tend to fluctuate on our health all the time, and it seems hard to always "be good." Sleep has a personality like a cat. It can be friendly and sweet, but it seems to be only on its terms. Sleep comes when it feels like it and almost always does not seem to obey your commands. New research has shown that cats may be more loyal than we think. Getting good sleep is both art and a science – even for people who have mastered every other aspect of their lives. This whole book has been a lot about finding that specific recipe that will fix your sleep. This chapter is a reminder that you, your state of mind and your sleep will evolve and change over time. Don't hesitate to restructure your recipe, keep it up to date and fresh for what you and your body need.

In Daniel Pink's book When, he has a chapter called "Avoid a False Start with a Premortem." A postmortem is when a coroner determines the cause of death. But a premortem gives us a chance to look at what will kill something. In the case of this program we want to look at what will cause you to fail. What you want to think about is what is going to be the thing that stops you from being successful. What will interrupt your sleep challenge? Why does the proverbial gym membership fail? Why will kill this sleep intervention? You know yourself, what will destroy your success at this. Own it. One example might be what Daniel refers to as the quest for the perfect start day. I think it does make a difference when you put a date on the calendar and plan to begin something new. For women, they will have a much better result in any diet or exercise plan if they begin it at the start of their menstrual month. At the start of a new month or a new week, set out a few days and allow time to truly lay out your plan. A plan isn't a plan without concrete effort being put in. Lack of sleep, as I have no doubt bored you with enough, is destructive to our will power and emotions. If you are trying to fix your sleep, you can't wing it and show up at bedtime hoping a house elf will deliver tea and massage you to sleep. Be your own grown-up and care for yourself as you would others.

Monday morning is perhaps the most important part of my week. It sets the tempo for what is to come. When I take the time to tidy the house, tidy my work plan, and think through what kid stuff, meals, and family commitments there are for the week, I feel better about the whole week. I also like to know my big rocks for the month and what else needs to happen. For me, this is Monday morning. You are about to have a Monday morning with a new routine and new habits. Have you put all the pieces in place to make that easy for yourself? I like to think about it as making your lunch the night before. You can plan to take those leftovers, but unless I take the time to put them in a container with the portion size for my lunch, it usually doesn't happen. Best-laid plans and all of that. I eat out and continue with my current bad habits. Planning is your friend. Set aside daily, weekly, and monthly times to clear the decks and evaluate how things are going. Ultimately, the success of this will fall not on you as a person but as a sum of your behaviors. Plant the seeds for success in this sleep garden and tend it like you want the vegetables in the end. You can't let weeds grow and never water; it won't work.

Another great book is the 5 Second Rule by Mel Robbins. She describes in her book that she found it difficult to get out of bed in the morning and that the snooze button on her alarm clock routinely won. But her rule has her and countless others, including myself, take back control of her life. She credits the countdown of 5, 4, 3, 2, 1 to launching her inner self. This mechanism activates your brain to focus on change. This rule is for when "you know you should do" something but feel hesitant. Think of it a countdown to jump off a cliff. You may use this when you lie down to meditate for the first time or when you go to start a conversation with your partner. I taught swimming lessons when I was a teenager, and I used the countdown to get kids to jump in the water when they were scared. Come on in, the water is warm – or maybe cool for deep sleep (bad joke, I know). Another favorite book is Eat That Frog, and yes, it is truly that. Brian Tracey encourages us to master the courage to eat the frogs during the day. Frogs are the tasks we don't want to do and just like the 5 Second Rule, you need to eat the biggest and ugliest frogs first. Do the 80/20 rule if you need to. Take the bull by the horns. Carpe diem.

Dogs can't resist stopping everything to chase a squirrel. Distractions are a problem for all of us. There are squirrels everywhere. I consistently tease Caleb that if a squirrel is a block away, just like our dog, he will get distracted. This plan encourages you to look at sleep holistically, and you may add interventions when you want because it is your plan. But breaking bad habits and forming new ones will take patience, time, and grit. Relapse, especially if you get sick or something unexpected happens, may derail you. Coming up with your own rule on how you should handle any squirrels is important. In the book Thinking Fast and Slow, Daniel Kahneman states that multitasking can be dangerous. When you are tired, you will not do the new habit or the extra habit. It will get dropped. I think about this as far as diet. It is easy to set out and start out, but then you end up with an expected business dinner and you end up falling off the wagon. It is okay. Fall off the wagon. But have a plan to get back on and what and how you will make that happen. This is not a strict plan, and there is room to wiggle. Use it if you need to, but it can't be an excuse. An excuse means you didn't try hard to solve the problem. No excuses; only solved problems.

Triggers are prompts and anchors for the interventions. When you anchor your new habits – or, even better, a habit you already do – to a block of time you make it easy for your brain to just group them and not set down a whole new set of tracks. Write down the plan and the trigger points together as well. Writing helps commit the plan to memory, and I feel like seeing it in black and white can also make it seem more real. Feel free to add potential squirrels and premortems as well. Write it all down. Damon Zahariades, in Morning Makeover, talks about choosing between the "freedom" of feeling like you can do whatever you want with no routine. But that generally isn't productive. When you have a list or plan for your morning, you actually get more done during the day. For you tech types, yes put it in a Word document or notes or set calendar reminders. If you were to go back to school and have to memorize all the countries of the world and their capitals, how would you do it? I bet you have a sense on what learner profile you are and how you might start that.

You cannot do this all by yourself. I am the queen of "I've got this." You may be a control freak and type A and all of that, but you probably don't sleep alone, work out alone, or have lunch breaks alone. If you are all alone for all of these things always, you need to read Belong by Radha Agrawal and get some help. No one should be alone. In a 2018 study, Matt Walker ties lack of sleep to individuals enforcing greater social separation from others. Don't let your sleep deprivation pull you away from others. Tell someone you are doing this, even if you just say, I need five hugs a day as part of my prescription for better sleep. Weight Watchers, AA, and other successful interventions need an accountability partner. I tried to write this book for two years. It was not until I signed up for an accountability partner and set unmovable deadlines that I took the plunge.

Jessica had to have a cohort in order to succeed. She needed the accountability. She is that person, the head of the PTA, Bible study, book club, church group – the social butterfly. Working one on one is good for the groundwork but she is a pack animal. She participates in run/walk events and is the person you want on your committee. Her motivation is helping others, and that means she takes other people on that amazing ride. If you are a Jessica, then you know that if you are "doing this to help someone else," then you will be way more motivated. If you have a Jessica in your life, then you are blessed. You have a cheerleader in your corner. Community doesn't naturally seem to be part of sleep. But setting goals for what you want to do with your sleep-superpowered life, that is worth sharing. Jessica tackled sleep with her walking buddies. She was tired of being tired and dragging as they walked. Turns out, they all were dragging. They did the "self-inventory" not by themselves but as a group. They were able to talk through what might work and laugh over the things they couldn't imagine doing. They shared what kept them up at night and what was preventing them from becoming their best selves. They were able to grow as friends and people. Health has to become more of a community and sharing activity. Doctors and hospitals are great for triage and extreme health problems, but sleep, diet, and exercise can all be helped a lot just by sharing with each other.

Don't Give Up

It is tempting to drop and disregard things that fail, especially after a few tries. Failure is almost certain for at least some of the things you are about to try. Research suggests it could take fifteen times before a baby will accept a new food, so the first few bites may be a bust. And if you know it is failing, try it with something that works. You are not so different from that baby. Sometimes we don't want to eat our vegetables, even if they are good for us. If you feel hesitant about the yoga nidra or magnesium, well, put on your big girl panties and suck it up. Document failures and do your best to objectively evaluate them before dismissing and pitching it off the highchair. You may discover that there is a complex web and stuff that is attaching to a failing intervention. Writing it down and dissecting it might allow you to untangle it a little.

Time is not the same for any of us. I so love the topic of time. I am super geeky, and as a physics nerd, I find it a treat to think about. I understand a lot of you are about to jump ship and start skimming, but you are already here, and this will only take a paragraphs' worth of your time. Your time is the point. Without getting all physics, time is a faulty variable. It is so subjective that time actually passes at a different rate at your head than at your feet. It is clearly demonstrated when we feel time differently based on the tasks we do. "A watched kettle never boils." Meditation, breath work, and stress breaks can seem like they are cutting into your time. But I challenge that thought. When you take the time, you need to be peaceful, to sleep, to balance, you will get time back in the form of productivity. Susan is a great example: she spends more time on sleep now, but is happier, more organized, and more productive with the rest of her time. Being sleep deprived is like slugging through mud. Time will slow down and tasks take more time and seem harder. Give time for this plan, your recipe, your sleep, and you will own your time.

Balance, expanding awareness, and some of the teachings of Ayurveda and TCM give us a different perspective on our health and wellness. But for most of us they may not makes sense. Some of the language and descriptions seem confusing. For example, sleep and insomnia are considered to be the imbalance of both heart and liver. An excess heat in the liver? Seems confusing and for our western minds a stretch to understand and implement. While many people have heard the term yin-yang or know its famous symbol, few understand what yin-yang truly is. In terms of the human body, yin is associated with the lower parts of the body, while yang is associated with the upper body and back. Given yin and yang's interconnectivity, diseases are not seen as entities separate from the body but instead are understood as states of yin and yang imbalance. Sleep and insomnia in both systems of treatments are about imbalance. Whether you decide to try some of the interventions from Eastern medicine is up to you. But recognition that you are trying to fix an imbalance, in your circadian rhythm and in your health, is big. Especially if the rest of your life seems pretty orderly now, rebalancing your health pendulum may shift other things too, until your pendulum stops swinging.

Change is stressful. Stress is something we have talked about in this book a lot. In those cases, we are talking about bad stress – the lion that actually isn't about to eat you, the guy who cut you off, but no-one was actually hurt.

This stress is toxic. But is it? In 1998, 30,000 adults in the United States were asked how much stress they had experienced in the previous year. The question was "Do you believe stress is bad for your health?" The results were released eight years later and included that 46 percent of respondents had died from high stress.[124] But the increase of stress wasn't the governing risk factor. It was the belief that stress is hurting your health that is the biggest factor. The perception of how you sleep will influence it.

When we track our sleep, often when you feel tired in the morning, we want to think that the night was a waste and we didn't get any sleep. Last night could have been that for me. I have too many book thoughts in my head and combined with noisy, late-night teenagers, my Oura ring said that I slept five hours. Well that sucks. Or does it? I do use my OOLER and the three bucket and mmm, and from all this, I actually got two hours of deep sleep and two hours of REM. My first response could have been, I know I didn't fall asleep until well after 1:00 and it wasn't a good night based on OURA's sleep score, lots of red lines. But reminding myself that I got what I needed for today settled out my emotional plunge. I didn't fail at sleep. I didn't get an A+. But I got what I need for today. I absolutely fall into the trap of putting pressure on my sleep, especially before a big talk, but I have never failed to deliver those talks. I must have gotten what I needed despite poor sleep.

Belief about our stress, our health, and our sleep is as important to the equation as what is actually going on. Mind over matter and the placebo effect are facts not fiction. Go back to your why: will you fail it because of a bad night's sleep? If the answer is no, then you got what you need.

---

[124] Keller, Abiola, et al. "Does the perception that stress affects health matter? The association with health and mortality." *Health psychology* 31.5 (2012): 677.

Fulfillment – feeling inspired and lifted up by our family, our community, our work, and our life – this is not something people are lucky to find. In Simon Sinek's book Find Your Why, he acknowledges that generalized terms like "find your passion," aren't enough to instantly give you fulfillment. There is actually a World Happiness Report that ranks 156 countries by happiness levels. I think that is kind of cool. In 2019, the top ten was again dominated by the Nordic countries, with Denmark, Norway, and Iceland taking the leading spots followed by the Netherlands, Switzerland, Sweden, New Zealand, Canada, and Austria. The United States dropped one place, to nineteenth. It is a country's social safety net combined with personal freedom and a good work-life balance that gives it an edge. Almost half of Finns donate regularly to charity, and almost a third said they had given up time to volunteer for a charity in the previous month. It is important to take your list of goals you get with your sleep superpowers and turn them into fulfillment. This is the ultimate why. Where is your why for sleep? It will be these whys that provide fulfillment and happiness when you are eating those frogs. For me, it's my kids. When I wanted to curl up in a ball and sit out the rest of my life after Benjamin died, it was them. They still needed me. Todd pulled me up off my knees as we left Benjamin for the last time, and he said just that: "Your other boys still need you." It was the why then, and it still is today. As they have gotten older, it is less about physically taking care of them and more about coaching, guiding, and providing a soft place to land. This is yours and yours alone. Put your why big in your day, in your gratitude, in front of you as you place the frog in your mouth. There should be nothing you wouldn't do for your why.

I love the word resilience.

According to the American Psychological Association, resilience is the process of adapting well in the face of adversity, trauma, tragedy, threats, or even significant sources of risk. In simple terms, we might describe resilience as the ability to bounce back when something goes wrong rather than crack under pressure[125]. The good news is that everyone has some resilience, only in varying degrees. It's important to note that a person with resilience still feels the intensity of a difficult situation – they've just found a better (and quicker) way of dealing with it. Fortunately, resilience can be learned, and not surprisingly, it can make or break your career.

Resilience has gotten you this far, despite the fact that you may be so sleep deprived you are like a drunk person wandering through life.

Courage is another power word. As you step out of your comfort zone and take control of sleep, you will use courage. You have used it to get out of bed and face another uphill day of being tired. But you need to dig deep and find the courage to get an accountability partner, show up ready with a plan, and stand up to your failures.

---

[125] Castrillon, Caroline. "Why Resilience Can Make Or Break Your Career." Forbes, *Forbes* Magazine, 16 Oct. 2019, www.forbes.com/sites/carolinecastrillon/2019/10/13 /why-resilience-can-make-or-break-your-career/#573afd5318e6.

CHAPTER 13

Awaken the Greatness within You

"Greatness is not measured by what a man or woman accomplishes, but by the opposition he or she has overcome to reach his goals."
— Dorothy Height —

Arthur C. Clarke, cowriter of *2001: A Space Odyssey*, put forth the following three laws. (It is okay if you are not a sci-fi geek like me, but these are just practical.)

1. When a respected scientist says something is possible, he is probably right. When he states something is impossible, he is probably wrong.

2. The only way to discover what is possible is to push past the current limits.

3. Any sufficiently advanced technology feels like magic.

I am going to put you in the role of the scientist from the first law. Do you think that great sleep is possible? Or impossible? Either way you are right, but who wants to be the naysayer in this case? Decide that it is possible. As you move your way around the track above, are you controlling and monitoring the thoughts that think this is possible? If you are all in, set a date and start, give yourself that goal you will do when you get this program done. If you approach this as an occasional approach, it will not work. This is an everyday plan. For thirty days, you must commit to yourself through sleep. Don't worry about diet or exercise; use your will power for sleep. Put stickie notes up, set out tea bags, make your bedroom a sleep room. You have all the tools to be successful if you don't buy them before you start, you won't have them there when you need them. If you were to train for a marathon you would need running shoes and a plan. Get your stuff together, and certainly don't start this before you have the equivalent of those running shoes. Eliminate your excuses before they happen. You know yourself better than anyone. You know what you will do to sabotage yourself. Did you point it out in the self-inventory? Don't become your enemy, be a good friend to yourself.

I gave birth naturally to all of my boys. Every single time as I was about to transition from pushing and the final phase, I wanted to give up. I am not alone. That is part of the process, and no matter how much you prepare, when you get to that moment, you are sure you can't keep doing this labor thing. It is like that in life too. It is darkest before the dawn. But remember that when you want to give up on this, it means you are about to see what you thought was impossible is possible.

I believe in pushing limits – not all of the time of course, but to occasionally get out of your comfort zone is good for you.

"Never despise small beginnings, and don't belittle your own accomplishments. Remember them and use them as inspiration as you go on to the next thing. When you venture outside your comfort zone, wherever the starting point may be, it's kind of a big deal."

– Chris Guillebeau –

This is your journey, your story, and the fork in your road. Let this be the moment that you start living. After the death of my son, I felt like my bubble burst, that the life I dreamed of, with the white picket fence, was destroyed. I still feel frustrated with my body, my weight, and what I feel like I have committed to stay healthy, but this is life. The bubble will burst for us all in different ways. You must decide what to do with what you are given. You must love yourself enough to say no to that glass of wine close to your bedtime. To turn to a walk or yoga or meditation to feel better and less stressed. You must decide when to take a drug and when to try a lifestyle intervention first.

You must recognize the foundational place that sleep and this program have for you and your optimized self. When you solve sleep this way instead of taking a pill, you are doing it the "hard" way, but you own all of it and the "side effect" of a healthy life is joy and a better quality of life.

Google just partnered with Big Pharma, so we see drugs as a solution everywhere. It is hard to avoid getting rolled over by drug companies with the allure of an instant fix. Opioids tell a different story of that fix for pain. There is no happily ever after commercial for the opioid crisis. When will we stop fooling ourselves that chronic problems can be fixed with an instant solution? CBT works better for pain and has better results in the long term. But the patient has to work at it: be involved, jump in with two feet. Diabetes treatments are making more progress than any drug trial with apps and interventions where the patient closes the feedback loop and can make decisions about their health for themselves in the moment. There is no list of side effects for deciding to make healthy choices. There are no downsides if you suddenly start meditating too much, give too many hugs, share your journey, or help people around you. Healing your sleep will inspire you to share and help people with this problem. It may inspire you to be healthier in other areas of your life. It may inspire you to share this habit of health with your kids.

Curing chronic pain, chronic insomnia, and autoimmune diseases is possible. But it isn't the easy way out. Creating new habits pushes you outside of your comfort zone, but studies confirm that doing something new and potentially frightening helps stave off burnout and is good for your brain. As you go through this first month of month of test and accept or test and discard, you change your brain for the better, on top of achieving your sleep superpowers.

I love the third law because I think it reminds us to be humble in our knowledge. Our science today, our smart life, would be magic and craziness to someone from 100, or even 50, years ago. Right now, people are starting to realize that sleep is critically important. People need to know that getting good sleep isn't magic; it is a process. You are the lead scientist in your experiment to prove getting sleep isn't magic. It is grounded in habits, our circadian rhythms, and respecting our relationships to each other and the planet. Hunter-gatherers worshiped the sun; it was the center of their lives. They slept on the ground and grounded themselves, perpetually. They connected with each other after a long day, slept in one big room and shared space. Exposure to the sun gives us vitamin D, and the sunlight that warms our faces tells our brains to produce serotonin. The rise and fall of the temperature during the day signals our core body temperature to change and sends us to restful deep sleep. Our modern, convenient life is failing our bodies. This is a chance to bring back the magic of sleep. Be a caveman or cavewoman and enjoy this beautiful planet and the herd of humans you live with and around.

Your knowledge of sleep from this book has been designed to answer your questions about sleep and give you that relaxed, "you've got this" confidence. Nothing in this book is rocket science. Trust me, I have done that; this is easier and harder at the same time. I love reading about, watching movies about, and learning almost anything about people who climb Mount Everest. The stories of survival in conditions where the planet is winning at trying to kill you seem extreme, but somedays it feels like my life is trying to kill me as well. Steven Kessler, in his book The 5 Personality Patterns, describes being present versus being in a pattern. Being present is just like it sounds and allows us to complete tasks and overcome. Being in a pattern means we are letting the past or personality quirks disrupt progress. We fall out of being present when we are hit by stress or some event that suddenly transports us into our pattern. Usually these patterns develop in childhood or when we survive something. But these survival patterns are not our actual selves; they are just what we fall into when the road seems bumpy.

I fell into a survival pattern when Benjamin died. I may have been in that pattern on and off previous to that event, but the impact of his death put me into survival. These patterns shape are perceptions of reality and usually limit what we can accomplish. When we suffer from insomnia for a long time, we are set in a survival sleep pattern. We deny our bodies further because most of us don't want to spend time and energy on things we fail at. There is a saying, "The beatings will continue until morale improves." Freud called this critic in our heads the "superego"; in childhood, it serves the purpose to get us to "be good." It can use shame and self-defamation to convince us we don't need one more cookie. But it is important to remind ourselves that this critic and our self-image when we are tired and depressed are not usually positive. We need to audit the inner voice. Protect this goal of sleep, because sleep gives you control over that voice.

When either my outer world or my inner world (and sometimes both) are trying to push me off course, I need to center. I think back to where we talked about your core values, who are you in that diamond center? I ground my thoughts, and sometimes physically ground my body to get rid of the electrical currents in my brain and body. I have since I was a child had a special bubble that I picture myself in. Especially at night, my bubble keeps all of the other "stuff" out. When I had kids, when they woke up at night, we would cuddle, and I pictured my bubble surrounding us; safe, quiet, and peaceful, we could fall asleep. Thoughts are crazy things. Inside our head, they all feel like they are us. The things we say to each other and to ourselves feel like they come from that person in our head. But when my boys were plagued with the hormones of puberty, I often heard thoughts come out that weren't them. The negative thoughts of depression are often because of hormone imbalance. Lack of sleep makes us grumpy. We can all picture that unruly child, up past his or her bedtime and agree that his or her thoughts and behaviors are not who that child is when he or she is rested. You are starting this journey tired and beaten down by sleep. Your thoughts may misbehave like that child. Set rules for your thoughts, ground yourself back to the purpose of your sleep quest.

The Evening Gatha (a Zen chant)
Let me respectfully remind you
Life and death are of supreme importance.
Time swiftly passes by and opportunity is lost.
Each of us should strive to awaken
Awaken.
Take heed.
This night, your days are diminished by one.
Do not squander your life.
Share, Make It Your Mission to Stop Insomnia

Helping people sleep and stopping people like me from going through their lives drunk is my passion. I hope this book has empowered you to find your sleep recipe. But my hope is you don't stop there. Sleep is desperately in need of ambassadors. I opened my TEDx talk with this:

"I did the equivalent of driving my kids to school drunk every day, and it didn't stand out; nobody jumped in, there was no outrage. Why? It is estimated that 50 percent of the world's population suffers from insomnia at least once a month. But we are keeping our insomnia a secret. No one is jumping up and down about this huge sleep problem. A study shows that moderate sleep deprivation produces impairments equivalent to those of alcohol intoxication. After seventeen to nineteen hours without sleep, performance was equivalent or worse than that of a blood alcohol concentration (BAC) level of 0.05 percent. If you miss a whole night's sleep it is 0.1 percent. Sleep deprivation is attached to mental illness and depression. No one, including me, is owning this insomnia problem. For more than a year, I consistently did not sleep through the night. I did my mom duties, worked, drove, and survived. But if I did this drunk, a friend, colleague, someone would have likely intervened. But insomnia is linked to every mental illness, and if you don't sleep, as we all know, we get angry, depressed, and frustrated more easily. We all know when our kids are tired when they are all those things, but we are not able to see our friends not sleeping and they suffer alone." I believe that since we don't have a sobriety test for insomnia that it forces people to suffer alone.

We are the power in the movement for sleep. Our smart, technology-driven world has put the power in our hands. We feel power shifting in the world dynamics. In Jeremy Heimann and Henry Timm's book, *New Power*, one of my current favorites by the way, they look at how the power is shifting from an old power view to a new power view. Both views are wrong. They confine us to a narrow debate about technology in which either everything is changing, or nothing is. In reality, a much more interesting and complex transformation is just beginning, one driven by a growing tension between two distinct forces: old power and new power. Old power is like currency or banks. The power is held by few and is doled out when they see fit. It is closed and hard to access. New power is like a river; it flows based on mass. It is open: jump in and swim along. I believe that the hospital and medical system today is old power. It diagnoses problems to guidelines it derives. It gives treatment as it sees fit. It created the opioid crisis with its power, and we, as the river, have to navigate around its pitfalls. The future is for health to be new power, held by the people. We can be part of the new power if we want. But new power isn't a spectator sport. You have to jump in and take control of your health – in this case, sleep. You are responsible for sharing it and passing the power on the others around you. In the book they talk about harnessing the three storms, taking human stories and creating urgency and building them into a movement. This is you today. Lack of sleep is an epidemic. Share your story and success; change the world through sleep. The sleep movement is full of tired people, so it isn't sexy or glamorous. This is not a pink breast cancer awareness competitor, but maybe when you get your sleep superpowers, you will give this movement some glamor. Sleep is grass roots; one person at a time owning their sleep, their health, their outcome; and passing that empowerment on to other people.

Morning Gatha

Waking up this morning I smile
Twenty-four band-new hours are before me
I vow to live fully present in every moment
And look upon all being with eyes of compassion.

Works of Interest

Bragazzi, N.L.; Guglielmi, O.; Garbarino, S. SleepOMICS: How Big Data Can Revolutionize Sleep Science. *Int. J. Environ. Res. Public Health* 2019, *16*, 291.

"Valerian Essential Oil – Valerianae Aetheroleum (Valeriana Officinalis)." *Herbal Reference*, 2019, herbalref.com/valerian-essential-oil-valerianae-aetheroleum-valeriana-officinalis/.

Kryger, Meir, et al. "Principles and Practice of Sleep Medicine." *PRINCIPLES AND PRACTICE OF SLEEP MEDICINE: EXPERT CONSULT – ONLINE AND PRINT, 5TH EDITION*, 2017, doi:10.1016/c2012-0-03543-0.

Youngstedt, Shawn D., et al. "Human Circadian Phase–Response Curves for Exercise." *The Journal of Physiology*, vol. 597, no. 8, 2019, pp. 2253–2268., doi:10.1113/jp276943.

Manzar, Md. Dilshad, et al. "Humidity and Sleep: a Review on Thermal Aspect." *Biological Rhythm Research*, vol. 43, no. 4, 2012, pp. 439–457., doi:10.1080/09291016.2011.597621.

Shahid, Azmeh, et al. "Munich Chronotype Questionnaire (MCTQ)." *STOP, THAT and One Hundred Other Sleep Scales*, 2011, pp. 245–247., doi:10.1007/978-1-4419-9893-4_58.

Ryan, Richard M., and Edward L. Deci. "On Happiness and Human Potentials: A Review of Research on Hedonic and Eudaimonic Well-Being." *Annual Review of Psychology*, vol. 52, no. 1, 2001, pp. 141–166., doi:10.1146/annurev.psych.52.1.141.

"Body Clock & Sleep." *National Sleep Foundation*, 2019, www.sleepfoundation.org/articles/sleep-drive-and-your-body-clock.

"Assess and Improve Your Sleep." *AAFP Home | American Academy of Family Physicians*, 16 July 2017, www.aafp.org/home.html.

Gannon, Megan. "Can Any Animals Survive Without Sleep?" *LiveScience*, Purch, 2 Mar. 2019, www.livescience.com/64873-can-animals-survive-without-sleep.html.

Saper, Clifford B. "Staying awake for dinner: hypothalamic integration of sleep, feeding, and circadian rhythms." *Progress in brain research* 153 (2006): 243-252.

Administrator."Oxidation-Reduction (Redox) Reactions." *Home*, 2019, www.veedhibadi.com/oxidation-reduction-redox-reactions.

Roberts, Gregory David. *Shantaram: a Novel*. Pan Macmillan Australia, 2015.

Anaclet, Christelle, et al. "The GABAergic parafacial zone is a medullary slow wave sleep–promoting center." *Nature neuroscience* 17.9 (2014): 1217.

Lee, Seung-Hee, and Yang Dan. "Neuromodulation of Brain States." *Neuron*, vol. 76, no. 1, 2012, pp. 209–222., doi:10.1016/j.neuron.2012.09.012.

Szymusiak, Ronald. "Body Temperature and Sleep." *Handbook of Clinical Neurology Thermoregulation: From Basic Neuroscience to*

Clinical Neurology Part I, 2018, pp. 341–351., doi:10.1016/b978-0-444-63912-7.00020-5.

Lewis, Philip, et al. "Exercise Time Cues (Zeitgebers) for Human Circadian Systems Can Foster Health and Improve Performance: a Systematic Review." *BMJ Open Sport & Exercise Medicine*, vol. 4, no. 1, 2018, doi:10.1136/bmjsem-2018-000443.

"How to Sleep Better." *HelpGuide.org*, 13 Nov. 2019, www.helpguide.org/articles/sleep/getting-better-sleep.htm.

de Zambotti, Massimiliano, et al. "The sleep of the ring: comparison of the ŌURA sleep tracker against polysomnography." *Behavioral sleep medicine* 17.2 (2019): 124-136.

Hare, Holly. "Lack of Sleep Is Killing Us, Experts Warn." *Orlando Sentinel*, 25 Sept. 2017.

Bach, Natasha. "Life Expectancy in the U.S. Is Down for the Second Year as Opioid Deaths Soar." *Fortune*, Fortune, 21 Dec. 2017, fortune.com/2017/12/21/us-life-expectancy-declines-for-second-year/.

Veehof, M. M., et al. "Acceptance- and Mindfulness-Based Interventions for the Treatment of Chronic Pain: a Meta-Analytic Review." *Cognitive Behaviour Therapy*, vol. 45, no. 1, 2016, pp. 5–31., doi:10.1080/16506073.2015.1098724.

Buettner, Dan. "Blue Zone Lessons." *Blue Zones*, 2019, www.bluezones.com/dan-buettner/.

"The Nobel Prize in Physiology or Medicine 2017." *NobelPrize.org*, 2 Oct. 2017, www.nobelprize.org/prizes/medicine/2017/press-release/.

Bei, Bei, et al. "Chronotype and Improved Sleep Efficiency Independently Predict Depressive Symptom Reduction after Group

Cognitive Behavioral Therapy for Insomnia." *Journal of Clinical Sleep Medicine*, 2015, doi:10.5664/jcsm.5018.

Vetter, Céline, et al. "Mismatch of Sleep and Work Timing and Risk of Type 2 Diabetes." *Diabetes Care*, vol. 38, no. 9, 2015, pp. 1707–1713., doi:10.2337/dc15-0302.

Manfredini, Roberto, et al. "Daylight Saving Time, Circadian Rhythms, and Cardiovascular Health." *Internal and Emergency Medicine*, vol. 13, no. 5, 2018, pp. 641–646., doi:10.1007/s11739-018-1900-4.

Nowack, Kati, and Elke Van Der Meer. "The Synchrony Effect Revisited: Chronotype, Time of Day and Cognitive Performance in a Semantic Analogy Task." *Chronobiology International*, vol. 35, no. 12, 2018, pp. 1647–1662., doi:10.1080/07420528.2018.150 0477.

Ingram, Krista K, et al. "Molecular Insights into Chronotype and Time-of-Day Effects on Decision-Making." *Scientific Reports*, vol. 6, no. 1, 8 July 2016, doi:10.1038/srep29392.

"The Costs of Insufficient Sleep." *RAND Corporation*, www.rand.org/randeurope/research/projects/the-value-of-the-sleep-economy.html.

Hogeback, Jonathan. "Why Are Flamingos Pink?" *Encyclopædia Britannica*, Encyclopædia Britannica, Inc., Dec. 2017, www.britannica.com/story/why-are-flamingos-pink.

Miller, Wc, et al. "A Meta-Analysis of the Past 25 Years of Weight Loss Research Using Diet, Exercise or Diet plus Exercise Intervention." *International Journal of Obesity*, vol. 21, no. 10, 21 Oct. 1997, pp. 941–947., doi:10.1038/sj.ijo.0800499

Morin, Amy. "7 Scientifically Proven Benefits Of Gratitude That Will Motivate You To Give Thanks Year-Round." *Forbes*, Forbes Magazine, 27 Nov. 2017, www.forbes.com/sites/amymorin/2014/11/23/7-scientifically-proven-benefits-of-gratitude-that-will-motivate-you-to-give-thanks-year-round/#2f932d5183c0.

Hill, Patrick L., et al. "Examining the Pathways between Gratitude and Self-Rated Physical Health across Adulthood." *Personality and Individual Differences*, vol. 54, no. 1, Jan. 2013, pp. 92–96., doi:10.1016/j.paid.2012.08.011.

Richard, Aline, et al. "Loneliness Is Adversely Associated with Physical and Mental Health and Lifestyle Factors: Results from a Swiss National Survey." *Plos One*, vol. 12, no. 7, 2017, doi:10.1371/journal.pone.0181442.

Crash Test Dummies. *Superman's Song*.

HOFF, BENJAMIN. *TAO OF POOH*. EGMONT Books LTD, 2003.

HOFF, BENJAMIN. *TE OF PIGLET*. EGMONT Books LTD, 2003.

Robinson, Elizabeth A. R., et al. "Six-Month Changes in Spirituality and Religiousness in Alcoholics Predict Drinking Outcomes at Nine Months*." *Journal of Studies on Alcohol and Drugs*, vol. 72, no. 4, 2011, pp. 660–668., doi:10.15288/jsad.2011.72.660.

Turner, Arlener D., et al. "Is Purpose in Life Associated with Less Sleep Disturbance in Older Adults?" *Sleep Science and Practice*, vol. 1, no. 1, 2017, doi:10.1186/s41606-017-0015-6.

Fromm, E. (1978-1979). Primary and secondary process in waking and in altered states of consciousness. *Journal of Altered States of Consciousness, 4*(2), 115–128.

Ryff, Carol D., and Burton Singer. "The Contours of Positive Human Health." *Psychological Inquiry*, vol. 9, no. 1, 1998, pp. 1–28., doi:10.1207/s15327965pli0901_1.

Ryff, Carol D., and Corey Lee M. Keyes. "The Structure of Psychological Well-Being Revisited." *Journal of Personality and Social Psychology*, vol. 69, no. 4, 1995, pp. 719–727., doi:10.1037//0022-3514.69.4.719.

"The Complex Relationship Between Sleep, Depression & Anxiety." *National Sleep Foundation*, 2017, www.sleepfoundation.org/excessive-sleepiness/health-impact/complex-relationship-between-sleep-depression-anxiety.

"The Sixteen Personality Types – High-Level." *The Personality Page*, 2019, www.personalitypage.com/high-level.html.

Jacobson E. The Technique of Progressive Relaxation. The Journal of Nervous and Mental Disease. 1924;60(6):568-578.

Team, Spine. "Why 'Pink Noise' Might Just Help You Get a Better Night's Sleep." *Health Essentials from Cleveland Clinic*, Health Essentials from Cleveland Clinic, 28 Oct. 2019, health.clevelandclinic.org/why-pink-noise-might-just-help-you-get-a-better-nights-sleep/.

Spielman AJ, Saskin P, Thorpy MJ. Sleep Restriction: A New Treatment of Insomnia. Sleep Res 1983; 12: 286.

A. Czeisler Charles, C. Zimmerman Janet, M. Ronda Joseph, C. Moore-Ede Martin, D. Weitzman Elliot, Timing of REM Sleep is Coupled to the Circadian Rhythm of Body Temperature in Man, *Sleep*, Volume 2, Issue 3, September 1980, Pages 329–346, https://doi.org/10.1093/sleep/2.3.329

Malla, S. S. (2013). Cross-cultural Validity of Ryff's Well-being Scale in India. *Asia-Pacific Journal of Management Research and Innovation*, *9*(4), 379–387. https://doi.org/10.1177/2319510X14523107

Administrator. *Downshifting Insomnia Blog*. 8 June 2008, downshiftingromania.blogspot.com/2008_06_01_archive.html.

Facer-Childs, Elise R., et al. "The Effects of Time of Day and Chronotype on Cognitive and Physical Performance in Healthy Volunteers." *Sports Medicine – Open*, vol. 4, no. 1, 2018, doi:10.1186/s40798-018-0162-z.

Paine, Sarah-Jane, et al. "The Epidemiology of Morningness/Eveningness: Influence of Age, Gender, Ethnicity, and Socioeconomic Factors in Adults (30-49 Years)." *Journal of Biological Rhythms*, vol. 21, no. 1, 2006, pp. 68–76., doi:10.1177/0748730405283154.

Barnes, Christopher M. "The Ideal Work Schedule, as Determined by Circadian Rhythms." *Harvard Business Review*, 28 Jan. 2015, hbr.org/2015/01/the-ideal-work-schedule-as-determined-by-circadian-rhythms.

Wilson, Clare. "The Illnesses Caused by a Disconnect between Brain and Mind." *New Scientist*, 3 Apr. 2019, www.newscientist.com/article/mg24232240-100-the-illnesses-caused-by-a-disconnect-between-brain-and-mind/.

Waterhouse, J., et al. "The Role of a Short Post-Lunch Nap in Improving Cognitive, Motor, and Sprint Performance in Participants with Partial Sleep Deprivation." *Journal of Sports Sciences*, vol. 25, no. 14, 2007, pp. 1557–1566., doi:10.1080/02640410701244983.

Aron, Jacob. "The World Is Getting Better, so Why Are We Convinced Otherwise?" *New Scientist*, 4 Sept. 2019, www.newscientist.com/article/mg24332460-900-the-world-is-getting-better-so-why-are-we-convinced-otherwise/.

Vitt, Laurie J., and Janalee P. Caldwell. "Thermoregulation, Performance, and Energetics." *Herpetology*, 2014, pp. 203–227., doi:10.1016/b978-0-12-386919-7.00007-1.

Cheshire, William P. "Autonomic Neuroscience: Basic and Clinical." *Autonomic Neuroscience*, vol. 105, no. 2, 2003, doi:10.1016/s1566-0702(03)00089-4.

Segran, Elizabeth. "The $70 Billion Quest for a Good Night's Sleep." *Fast Company*, Fast Company, 29 Apr. 2019, www.fastcompany.com/90340280/the-70-billion-quest-for-a-good-nights-sleep.

Schlossberg, Michael. "This Is How Depression & Sleep Trouble Are Related.", 18 July 2018, mikeschlossbergauthor.com/2018/07/19/this-is-how-depression-sleep-trouble-are-related/.

Pigeon W.R., Park H., Sateia M.J. (2006) Sleep and Pain. In: Sleep and Sleep Disorders. Springer, Boston, MA

Schneider, Nicole. "NLP for Better Sleep." *Global NLP Training Blog*, 27 Dec. 2015, www.globalnlptraining.com/blog/nlp-better-sleep/.

Lynch, Julie, and Charlotte E. Wilson. "Exploring the Impact of Choral Singing on Mindfulness." *Psychology of Music*, vol. 46, no. 6, 2017, pp. 848–861., doi:10.1177/0305735617729452.

Reyner, Luise A., and James A. Horne. "Suppression of Sleepiness in Drivers: Combination of Caffeine with a Short Nap." *Psychophysiology*, vol. 34, no. 6, 1997, pp. 721–725., doi:10.1111/j.1469-8986.1997.tb02148.x.

Wingard, Jessie. "Does Drinking Hot Drinks on a Scorching Summer's Day Really Cool You down?: DW: 25.07.2013." *DW.COM*, 25 July 2013,

Vanecek, Nikki. "Beating drowsiness without the stress." *TCM Acupuncture Clinic*, 2013, tcmwellnessclinic.com/.

Chabris, Christopher F., and Daniel J. Simons. *The Invisible Gorilla: and Other Ways Our Intuitions Deceive Us*. MJF Books, 2012.

Uzer, Sara. "7 Ways Self-Reflection And Introspection Will Give You A Happier Life." *Elite Daily*, 6 Mar. 2015, www.elitedaily.com/life/7-ways-self-reflection-introspection-will-give-happier-life/943309

Administrator. "The Most Accurate Sleep and Activity Tracker." *Oura Ring*, 2019, www.ouraring.com/.

Aili, Katarina, et al. "Reliability of Actigraphy and Subjective Sleep Measurements in Adults: The Design of Sleep Assessments." *Journal of Clinical Sleep Medicine*, vol. 13, no. 01, 2017, pp. 39–47., doi:10.5664/jcsm.6384.

Goyal, M, et al. "Meditation Programs for Psychological Stress and Well-Being: A Systematic Review and Meta-Analysis." *Deutsche Zeitschrift Für Akupunktur*, vol. 57, no. 3, 2014, pp. 26–27., doi:10.1016/j.dza.2014.07.007.

Hölzel, Britta K., et al. "Mindfulness Practice Leads to Increases in Regional Brain Gray Matter Density." *Psychiatry Research: Neuroimaging*, vol. 191, no. 1, 2011, pp. 36–43., doi:10.1016/j.pscychresns.2010.08.006.

Stephen Parker, Swami Veda Bharati, and Manuel Fernandez (*2013*) Defining Yoga-Nidra: Traditional Accounts, Physiological

Research, and Future Directions. International Journal of Yoga Therapy: 2013, Vol. 23, No. 1, pp. 11-16.

DeNoon, Daniel J. "Sleeping Pills Called 'as Risky as Cigarettes.'" *WebMD*, WebMD, 27 Feb. 2012, www.webmd.com/sleep-disorders/news/20120227/sleeping-pills-called-as-risky-as-cigarettes#1.

Kripke, Daniel F., et al. "Mortality Related to Actigraphic Long and Short Sleep." *Sleep Medicine*, vol. 12, no. 1, 2011, pp. 28–33., doi:10.1016/j.sleep.2010.04.016.

Sullivan, Meg. "Our Ancestors Probably Didn't Get 8 Hours a Night, Either." *UCLA*, UCLA, 15 Oct. 2015, newsroom.ucla.edu/releases/our-ancestors-probably-didnt-get-8-hours-a-night-either.

Barnes, Zahra. "Magnesium, the Invisible Deficiency That Hurts Health." *CNN*, Cable News Network, 3 Jan. 2015, www.cnn.com/2014/12/31/health/magnesium-deficiency-health/.

Gominak, S.c., and W.e. Stumpf. "The World Epidemic of Sleep Disorders Is Linked to Vitamin D Deficiency." *Medical Hypotheses*, vol. 79, no. 2, 2012, pp. 132–135., doi:10.1016/j.mehy.2012.03.031.

Brutto, Oscar H. Del, et al. "Dietary Fish Intake and Sleep Quality: a Population-Based Study." *Sleep Medicine*, vol. 17, 2016, pp. 126–128., doi:10.1016/j.sleep.2015.09.021.

DerSarkissian, Carol. "Sleep Deprivation and Memory Loss." *WebMD*, WebMD, 7 Aug. 2019, www.webmd.com/sleep-disorders/sleep-deprivation-effects-on-memory#1.

"Decreased Deep Sleep Linked to Early Signs of Alzheimer's Disease." *ScienceDaily*, ScienceDaily, 9 Jan. 2019, www.sciencedaily.com/releases/2019/01/190109142704.htm.

"The Costs of Insufficient Sleep." *RAND Corporation*, www.rand. org/randeurope/research/projects/the-value-of-the-sleep-economy. html.

Narcisse, Evan. "20,000 Per Cell: Why Midi-Chlorians Suck." *Time*, Time, 10 Aug. 2010, techland.time.com/2010/08/10/20000-per-cell-why-midi-chlorians-suck/.

"Refueling Your Energy Levels." *Harvard Health*, Harvard Health Publishing , Oct. 2018, www.health.harvard.edu/staying-healthy/ refueling-your-energy-levels.

Scullin, Michael K., and Donald L. Bliwise. "Sleep, Cognition, and Normal Aging." *Perspectives on Psychological Science*, vol. 10, no. 1, 2015, pp. 97–137., doi:10.1177/1745691614556680.

Hicklin, Tianna. "Molecular Ties between Lack of Sleep and Weight Gain." *National Institutes of Health*, U.S. Department of Health and Human Services, 22 Mar. 2016, www.nih.gov/news-events/nih-research-matters/molecular-ties-between-lack-sleep-weight-gain.

"The Complex Relationship Between Sleep, Depression & Anxiety." *National Sleep Foundation*, www.sleepfoundation.org/ excessive-sleepiness/health-impact/complex-relationship-be-tween-sleep-depression-anxiety.

Bhandari, Tamara. "Decreased Deep Sleep Linked to Early Signs of Alzheimer's Disease." *ScienceDaily*, ScienceDaily, 9 Jan. 2019, www.sciencedaily.com/releases/2019/01/190109142704.htm.

Onton, Julie A et al. "In-Home Sleep Recordings in Military Veterans With Posttraumatic Stress Disorder Reveal Less REM and Deep Sleep <1 Hz." *Frontiers in human neuroscience* vol. 12 196. 11 May. 2018, doi:10.3389/fnhum.2018.00196

Sun, Zhi-cheng, et al. "Extremely Low Frequency Electromagnetic Fields Facilitate Vesicle Endocytosis by Increasing Presynaptic Calcium Channel Expression at a Central Synapse." *Nature News*, Nature Publishing Group, 18 Feb. 2016, www.nature.com/articles/srep21774.

Becker, Robert O.,Marino, Andrew A.. *Electromagnetic forces and life processes*. Technology Review. 1972:32–38.

Cao, Honglong, et al. "Circadian Rhythmicity of Antioxidant Markers in Rats Exposed to 1.8 GHz Radiofrequency Fields." *International Journal of Environmental Research and Public Health*, vol. 12, no. 2, 2015, pp. 2071–2087., doi:10.3390/ijerph120202071.

Hutter, H-P. "Subjective Symptoms, Sleeping Problems, and Cognitive Performance in Subjects Living near Mobile Phone Base Stations." *Occupational and Environmental Medicine*, vol. 63, no. 5, 2006, pp. 307–313., doi:10.1136/oem.2005.020784.

Nickolaenko, A. P., and M. Hayakawa. *Resonances in the Earth-Ionosphere Cavity*. Springer, 2011.

Cherry, Neil. "Schumann Resonances, a Plausible Biophysical Mechanism for the Human Health Effects of Solar/Geomagnetic Activity." *Natural Hazards*, vol. 26, no. 3, 2002, pp. 279–331., doi:10.1023/a:1015637127504.

Pelka, Rainer B., et al. "Impulse Magnetic-Field Therapy for Insomnia: A Double-Blind, Placebo-Controlled Study." *Advances in Therapy*, vol. 18, no. 4, 2001, pp. 174–180., doi:10.1007/bf02850111.

Chevalier, Gaétan et al. "Earthing: health implications of reconnecting the human body to the Earth's surface electrons." *Journal of environmental and public health* vol. 2012 (2012): 291541. doi:10.1155/2012/291541

Cao, Huijuan et al. "Acupuncture for treatment of insomnia: a systematic review of randomized controlled trials." *Journal of alternative and complementary medicine (New York, N.Y.)* vol. 15,11 (2009): 1171-86. doi:10.1089/acm.2009.0041

Hof, Wim. "The History Of The 'Iceman' Wim Hof: Wim Hof Method." *The History Of The 'Iceman' Wim Hof | Wim Hof Method*, 2019, www.wimhofmethod.com/iceman-wim-hof.

Shevchuk, Nikolai A. "Adapted Cold Shower as a Potential Treatment for Depression." *Medical Hypotheses*, vol. 70, no. 5, 2008, pp. 995–1001., doi:10.1016/j.mehy.2007.04.052.

Harvard Health Publishing. "Anxiety and Stress Weighing Heavily at Night? A New Blanket Might Help." *Harvard Health*, Mar. 2019, www.health.harvard.edu/mind-and-mood/anxiety-and-stress-weighing-heavily-at-night-a-new-blanket-might-help.

Esmonde-White, Miranda. *Aging Backwards: Fast Track: 6 Ways in 30 Days to Look and Feel Younger.* HarperWave, an Imprint of HarperCollins Publishers, 2019.

Pradas, Jevan. *The Awakened Ape: a Biohacker's Guide to Evolutionary Fitness, Natural Ecstasy, and Stress-Free Living.* Tantor Media, 2018.

Dispenza, Joe, and Daniel G. Amen. *Breaking the Habit of Being Yourself: How to Lose Your Mind and Create a New One.* Hay House, 2015.

Kshirsagar, Suhas G., et al. *Change Your Schedule, Change Your Life: How to Harness the Power of Clock Genes to Lose Weight, Optimize Your Workout, and Finally Get a Good Night's Sleep.* Harper Wave, an Imprint of HarperCollinsPublishers, 2019.

Panda, Satchin. *The Circadian Code: Lose Weight, Supercharge Your Energy, and Tranform Your Health from Morning to Midnight.* Rodale, an Imprint of the Crown Publishing Group, 2018.

G. Egger, J. DixonBeyond obesity and lifestyle: a review of 21st century chronic disease determinants

Biomed Res Int, 2014 (2014), Article 731685

Y. Guo, A. Gasparrini, B. Armstrong, S. Li, *et al.*Global variation in the effects of ambient temperature on mortality: a systematic evaluation

Epidemiology, 25 (2014), pp. 781-789

Whole-body hyperthermia for the treatment of major depressive disorder: a randomized clinical trial

JAMA Psychiatry, 73 (2016), pp. 789-795

M.P. MattsonWhat doesn't kill you

Sci Amer, 313 (1) (2015), pp. 40-45

M.P. MattsonChallenging oneself intermittently to improve health

Dose-Resp, 12 (2014), pp. 600-618

M.P. Mattson, D.B. Allison, L. Fontana, M. Harvie, *et al.*Meal frequency and timing in health and disease

Proc Natl Acad Sci USA, 111 (2014), pp. 16647-16653

S.I.S. Rattan, R.A. Fernandes, D. Demirovic, B. Dymek, C.F. Lima-Heat stress and hormetin-induced hormesis in human cells: effects on aging, wound healing, angiogenesis, and differentiation

Dose-Resp, 7 (2008), pp. 90-103

Dehaene, Stanislas. *Consciousness and the Brain Deciphering How the Brain Codes Our Thoughts*. Viking, 2014.

Currey, Mason. *Daily Rituals: How Artists Work*. Alfred A. Knopf, 2016.

Milham, Samuel. *Dirty Electricity: Electrification and the Diseases of Civilization*. IUniverse, 2012.

Starr, Michelle. "Cats Bond Securely to Their Humans Maybe Even More Than Dogs Do." *ScienceAlert*, 23 Sept. 2019, www.sciencealert.com/cats-bond-securely-to-their-humans-maybe-even-more-than-dogs-do.

Robbins, Mel. *The 5 Second Rule: Transform Your Life, Work, and Confidence with Everyday Courage*. Savio Republic, 2017.

Simon, Eti Ben, and Matthew P. Walker. "Sleep Loss Causes Social Withdrawal and Loneliness." *Nature Communications*, vol. 9, no. 1, 2018, doi:10.1038/s41467-018-05377-0.

Moran, Tim P., and Jason S. Moser. "The Color of Anxiety: Neurobehavioral Evidence for Distraction by Perceptually Salient Stimuli in Anxiety." *Cognitive, Affective, & Behavioral Neuroscience*, vol. 15, no. 1, 2014, pp. 169–179., doi:10.3758/s13415-014-0314-7.

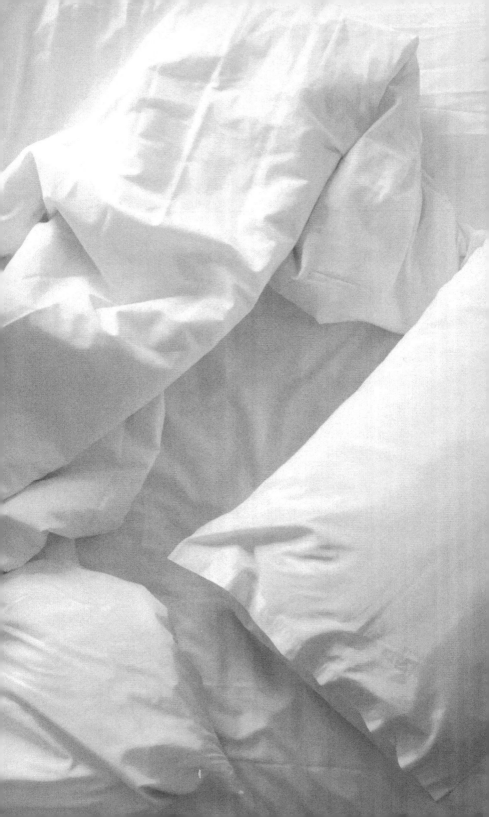

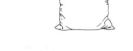

Sleep Worksheet

SLEEP IMPROVEMENT

Month of _____

RATE YOUR SLEEP, EVERY MORNING

M	T	W	T	F	S	S
○	○	○	○	○	○	○
○	○	○	○	○	○	○
○	○	○	○	○	○	○
○	○	○	○	○	○	○
○	○	○	○	○	○	○

:) :| :(

I RECOMMEND FILLING THE CIRCLES WITH HAPPY,
NEUTRAL OR SAD FACES.

DAILY HABITS EXAMPLE

Month of _____

START DAY WITH EXERCISE/OUTSIDE TIME							NO CAFFIENE AFTER 2 PM							GET YOUR DEEP WORK DONE IN THE MORNING						
M	T	W	T	F	S	S	M	T	W	T	F	S	S	M	T	W	T	F	S	S
○	○	○	○	○	○	○	○	○	○	○	○	○	○	○	○	○	○	○	○	○
○	○	○	○	○	○	○	○	○	○	○	○	○	○	○	○	○	○	○	○	○
○	○	○	○	○	○	○	○	○	○	○	○	○	○	○	○	○	○	○	○	○
○	○	○	○	○	○	○	○	○	○	○	○	○	○	○	○	○	○	○	○	○
○	○	○	○	○	○	○	○	○	○	○	○	○	○	○	○	○	○	○	○	○

BEDTIME HABITS EXAMPLE

Month of _____

CHANGE YOUR TEMPERATURE (TAKE A WALK, SHOWER, USE YOUR CHILIPAD)							REDUCE STRESS (MEDITATE, GRATITUDE, YOGA)							AS YOU GET IN BED... START THE DREAM YOU WANT TO HAVE...						
M	T	W	T	F	S	S	M	T	W	T	F	S	S	M	T	W	T	F	S	S
○	○	○	○	○	○	○	○	○	○	○	○	○	○	○	○	○	○	○	○	○
○	○	○	○	○	○	○	○	○	○	○	○	○	○	○	○	○	○	○	○	○
○	○	○	○	○	○	○	○	○	○	○	○	○	○	○	○	○	○	○	○	○
○	○	○	○	○	○	○	○	○	○	○	○	○	○	○	○	○	○	○	○	○
○	○	○	○	○	○	○	○	○	○	○	○	○	○	○	○	○	○	○	○	○

NIGHTTIME EXAMPLE

Month of _____

COOL DOWN IF YOU WAKE UP BEFORE THE MIDDLE OF THE NIGHT							WARM UP IF YOU WAKE EARLY OR DO MORE EXERCISES TO SETTLE YOUR MIND							BREATHING, YOGA, MEDITATION						
M	T	W	T	F	S	S	M	T	W	T	F	S	S	M	T	W	T	F	S	S
○	○	○	○	○	○	○	○	○	○	○	○	○	○	○	○	○	○	○	○	○
○	○	○	○	○	○	○	○	○	○	○	○	○	○	○	○	○	○	○	○	○
○	○	○	○	○	○	○	○	○	○	○	○	○	○	○	○	○	○	○	○	○
○	○	○	○	○	○	○	○	○	○	○	○	○	○	○	○	○	○	○	○	○
○	○	○	○	○	○	○	○	○	○	○	○	○	○	○	○	○	○	○	○	○

SLEEP PLAN DIARY

Month of _____

DID I FOLLOW MY DAYTIME TIPS?								DID I FOLLOW MY BEDTIME TIPS?								DID I SLEEP THROUGH MY DEEP SLEEP BUCKET?								DID I SLEEP UNTIL MY OPTIMAL WAKE UP TIME?						
M	T	W	T	F	S	S		M	T	W	T	F	S	S		M	T	W	T	F	S	S		M	T	W	T	F	S	S
○	○	○	○	○	○	○		○	○	○	○	○	○	○		○	○	○	○	○	○	○		○	○	○	○	○	○	○
○	○	○	○	○	○	○		○	○	○	○	○	○	○		○	○	○	○	○	○	○		○	○	○	○	○	○	○
○	○	○	○	○	○	○		○	○	○	○	○	○	○		○	○	○	○	○	○	○		○	○	○	○	○	○	○
○	○	○	○	○	○	○		○	○	○	○	○	○	○		○	○	○	○	○	○	○		○	○	○	○	○	○	○
○	○	○	○	○	○	○		○	○	○	○	○	○	○		○	○	○	○	○	○	○		○	○	○	○	○	○	○

NOTES _____

SLEEP IMPROVEMENT

Month of _____

RATE YOUR SLEEP, EVERY MORNING

M	T	W	T	F	S	S
○	○	○	○	○	○	○
○	○	○	○	○	○	○
○	○	○	○	○	○	○
○	○	○	○	○	○	○
○	○	○	○	○	○	○

☺   ☺   ☹

SELF INVENTORY EXAMPLE

	RATE HOW IMPORTANT THESE THINGS ARE TO YOU						
BEDTIME ENVIRONMENT	IMPORTANT		SOMEWHAT IMPORTANT		DOESN'T MATTER		
LIGHT	◯	◯	◯	◯	◯	◯	◯
SOUND	◯	◯	◯	◯	◯	◯	◯
TEMPERATURE	◯	◯	◯	◯	◯	◯	◯
BEDMATE/PETS/KIDS OTHER	◯	◯	◯	◯	◯	◯	◯
IS IT RELAXING OR STRESSFUL?	◯	◯	◯	◯	◯	◯	◯

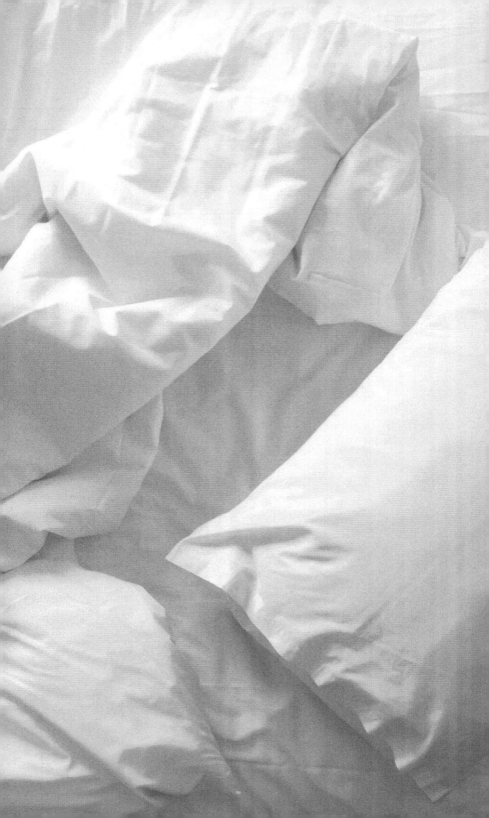

Chronotype Quiz

You have to do two hours of physically hard work. If you were entirely free to plan your day, in which of the following periods would you choose to do the work?

8:00 a.m. – 10:00 a.m. (4 points)
11:00 a.m. – 1:00 p.m. (3 points)
3:00 p.m. – 5:00 p.m. (2 points)
7:00 p.m. – 9:00 p.m. (1 point)

You have to take a two-hour test. You know it will be mentally exhausting. If you were entirely free to choose, when would you choose to take the test?

8:00 a.m. – 10:00 a.m. (4 points)
11:00 a.m. – 1:00 p.m. (3 points)
3:00 p.m. – 5:00 p.m. (2 points)
7:00 p.m. – 9:00 p.m. (1 point)

A friend has asked you to join him twice per week for a workout. The best time for him is between 10 p.m. and 11 p.m. With nothing else in mind other than how you normally feel in the evening, how do you think you would perform?

Very poorly (4 points)
Poorly (3 points)
Well enough (2 points)
Very well (1 point)

We hear about "morning" and "evening" types of people. Which of these types do you consider yourself?

Definitely morning type (6 points)
More a morning than an evening type (4 points)
More an evening than a morning type (2 points)
Definitely an evening type (0 points)

Add your scores together to get your total and compare your score with the table below to identify your chronotype.

Points	Type
1416 –	Definitely morning type
1113 –	Moderately morning type
910 –	Neither type
48 –	Moderately evening type
03 –	Definitely evening type

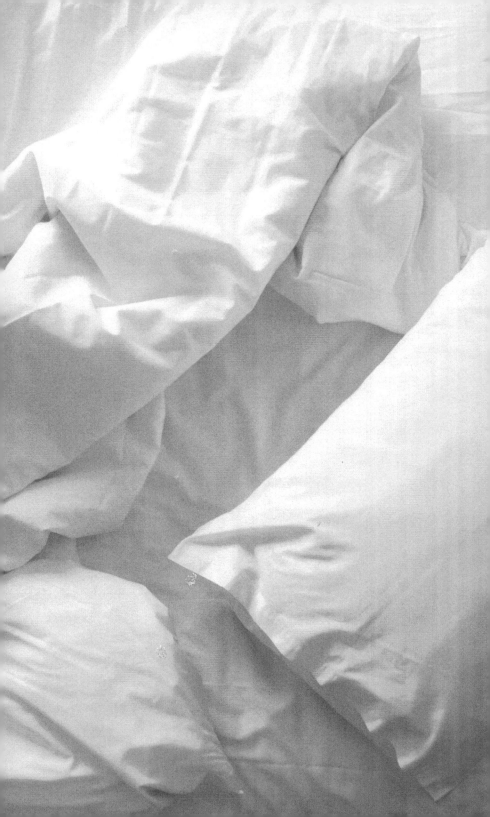

Possible Sleep/Day
Schedules

Morning Person

Time	Activity	Focus
6:00 a.m.	Wake-up	How was your sleep?
7:00-9:00 a.m.	Exercise/ go outside	Set intention for the day
9:00-12:00 a.m.	Productivity	Best time for deep work
12:00-1:00 p.m.	Lunch	Get outside/be healthy
1:00-5:00 p.m.	Afternoon productivity	Be creative
5:00-6:30 p.m.	Move, eat, connect	Leave work behind
6:30-9:00 p.m.	Connect, be outside	De stress
9:00-10:00 p.m.	Bedtime	Change your stress and temperature
10:00-3:00 a.m.	Deep Sleep	Stay cool for this sleep
3:00-6:00 a.m.	REM sleep	Warmer sleep

Middle Chronotype/ Lucky Ducks

Time	Activity	Focus
7:00 a.m.	Wake-up	How was your sleep?
8:00-10:00 a.m.	Exercise/ go outside	Set intention for the day
10:00-1:00 p.m.	Productivity	Best time for deep work
1:00-2:00 p.m.	Lunch	Get outside/be healthy
2:00-6:00 p.m.	Afternoon productivity	Be creative
6:00-7:30 p.m.	Move, eat, connect	Leave work behind
7:30-10:00 p.m.	Connect, be outside	De stress
10:00-11:00 p.m.	Bedtime	Change your stress and temperature
11:00-4:00 a.m.	Deep Sleep	Stay cool for this sleep
4:00-7:00 a.m.	REM sleep	Warmer sleep

Night Owls

Time	Activity	Focus
8:00 a.m.	Wake-up	How was your sleep?
9:00-10:00 a.m.	go outside	Set intention for the day

10:00-2:00 p.m.	Productivity	Best time for deep work
2:00-3:00PM	Lunch	Get outside/be healthy
3:00-4:00 p.m.	Nap	Get some extra sleep
4:00-6:30 p.m.	Afternoon productivity	Be creative
6:30-8:00 p.m.	Move, exercise, eat	Leave work behind
8:00-11:00 p.m.	Connect, relax	De stress
11:00-12:00 a.m.	Bedtime	Change your temperature
12:00-5:00 a.m.	Deep Sleep	Stay cool for this sleep
5:00-8:00 a.m.	REM sleep	Warmer sleep

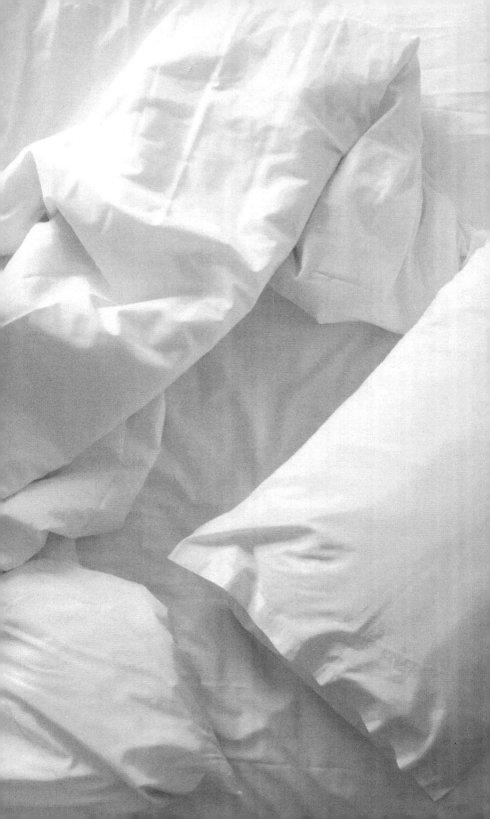

Thank You

Thank you so much for reading Reprogram Your Sleep: The Sleep Recipe that Works. If you've made it this far, I know one of two things about you. First, you're more ready than ever to leave your comfort zone where you do not sleep and second step out to embrace sleeping again.

I would love to learn more about your journey and success in conquering your sleep. Please keep in touch (I'm most active Facebook and Instagram), share your wins (tag me and use #Sleep-Geek), and visit ChiliTechnology.com for more resources, or send me an email at help@SleepGeek.me.

I'm passionate about stopping the sleep epidemic – not with drugs, but with higher consciousness and IQ about how sleep works. Part of the income from this book and my other programs go to this cause. Thanks in advance for helping me to take back sleep and making it accessible to everyone.

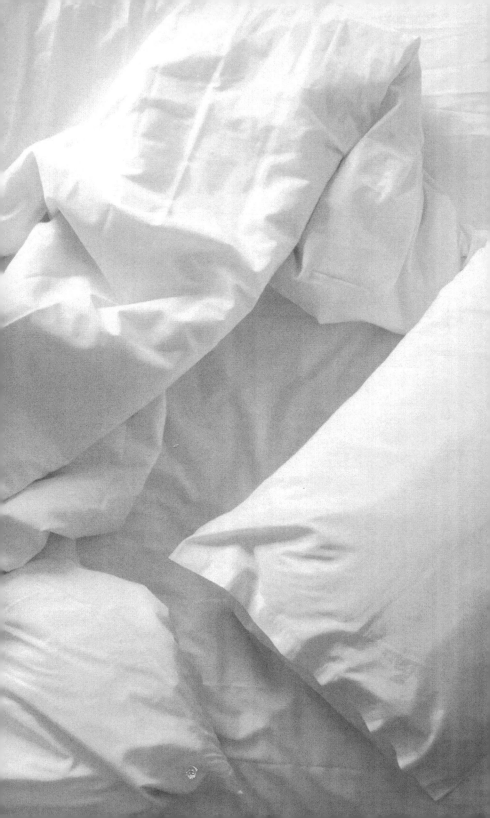

About the Author

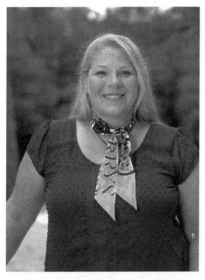

After the death of her son in 2008, Tara Youngblood suffered from insomnia and depression. Determined to find her way out, she spent over 10,000 hours studying the science of sleep. Applying her analytical skills from her physics and engineering background, combining multiple disciplines – including alternative medicine, and sleep diagnostics – her research led to a solution and over a dozen patent filings.

Tara now works with leading international researchers to further studies on sleep and explore ways to make sleep easier. She has connected over seventy research papers to the effects of temperature and sleep quality as the basis for over a dozen patents and sleep studies.

As co-founder and executive, she contributes to the strategic direction and daily operations of Chili Sleep Products As an expert in sleep science, Tara is a highly regarded international speaker. She is a seasoned entrepreneur with market-leading ingenuity and the ability to identify market opportunities. She and her husband,

Todd, have made multiple successful exits from ventures founded over the past twenty years.

Born in Alberta, Canada, she is a passionate global traveler, with visits to five continents and over a dozen countries. She is involved with multiple community philanthropic activities, including youth sports and international relief trips. Tara lives in Mooresville, North Carolina with her husband, Todd, four boys, a dog, three cats, and a rabbit. She loves the beach, mountains, almost anywhere outside.

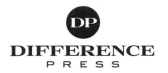

About Difference Press

Difference Press is the exclusive publishing arm of The Author Incubator, an educational company for entrepreneurs – including life coaches, healers, consultants, and community leaders – looking for a comprehensive solution to get their books written, published, and promoted. Its founder, Dr. Angela Lauria, has been bringing to life the literary ventures of hundreds of authors-in-transformation since 1994.

A boutique-style self-publishing service for clients of The Author Incubator, Difference Press boasts a fair and easy-to-understand profit structure, low-priced author copies, and author-friendly contract terms. Most importantly, all of our #incubatedauthors maintain ownership of their copyright at all times.

Let's Start a Movement with Your Message

In a market where hundreds of thousands of books are published every year and are never heard from again, The Author Incubator is different. Not only do all Difference Press books reach Amazon bestseller status, but all of our authors are actively changing lives and making a difference.

Since launching in 2013, we've served over 500 authors who came to us with an idea for a book and were able to write it and get it self-published in less than 6 months. In addition, more than 100 of those books were picked up by traditional publishers and are now available in book stores. We do this by selecting the highest quality and highest potential applicants for our future programs.

Our program doesn't only teach you how to write a book – our team of coaches, developmental editors, copy editors, art directors, and marketing experts incubate you from having a book idea to being a published, bestselling author, ensuring that the book you create can actually make a difference in the world. Then we give you the training you need to use your book to make the difference in the world, or to create a business out of serving your readers.

Are You Ready to Make a Difference?

You've seen other people make a difference with a book. Now it's your turn. If you are ready to stop watching and start taking massive action, go to http://theauthorincubator.com/apply/.

"Yes, I'm ready!"

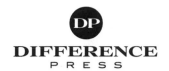

DIFFERENCE
P R E S S

Other Books by Difference Press

The Top 1% Life: The Real Estate Agent's Guide
to Free Up Your Time, Build Your Business with
Confidence, and Finally, Have a Life Outside of Sales!
by Kathleen Black

Get Back to Living: Navigating Through
the Loss of Your Spouse
by Allison L. Brown

Stop Worrying about Your Anxious Child: How
to Manage Your Child's Anxiety so You Can Finally Relax
by Tonya C. Crombie, Ph.D.

Become a Badass Rebel Runner: The Ultimate Guide
to Being a Fit Mom without the Diet Bullshit
by Jane Elizabeth

From Borderline to Baseline: 9 Key Steps
to Manage Your BPD and Start Loving Your Life
by Julie Ann Ford

Stop Draining Your Energy: The Movement Teacher's
Guide to Attract Clients You Love
by Heather Glidden

Is This Sickness or an Energy Block?:
Know the Difference and What to Do about It
by Amy Keast

Should I Leave My Relationship or Not?:
The Smart Woman's Guide to a Clear Path Forward
by Karen Lin

Side Hustle to Main Hustle: The Corporate Woman's
Guide to Full-Time Entrepreneurship
by Angel N. Livas

The Spiritual Entrepreneur: Quantum Leap
Into Your Next Level of Impact and Abundance
by Angelina Lombardo

Invention Protection Strategies: Expose
Your Intellectual Property and Fund Your Startup
by Cynthia Lombardo

Reverse Heart Disease Naturally: The Woman's Guide
to Not Die before Your Time
by Laurie Morse

Know What You Want Next: Break Free of the
'I Don't Know' Trap and Love Your Life Again
by Kimberly Napier

Build Your Business with Social Media:
The Step-by-Step Guide to Create a Life You Love
by Gry Sinding

Should I Leave Nursing?: 7 Steps to Career Clarity
by Karen Beck Wade, Ph.D.